7th Edition

THE ULTIMATE MELALEUCA GUIDE

Recommended uses for Melaleuca products based on research and the clinical experiences of health care professionals and veterinarians
AND
Proven household solutions recommended by people who use Melaleuca products every day

For more Melaleuca information, visit our website, **www.rmbarry.com**

1(888) 209-0510

PLEASE NOTE: It is recommended that you develop a good relationship with a physician knowledgeable in the art and science of natural and preventive medicine. The information in this book is not a substitute for the care you should be receiving from your primary physician. In all cases involving a physical or medical complaint, please consult your physician.

This book is intended to supply educational information to users of products manufactured by Melaleuca, Inc. It should not be used as sales literature or for business promotion.

All product names in this book (in italics) are registered trademarks of Melaleuca, Inc. of Idaho Falls, Idaho.

Published by:

RM Barry Publications
P.O. Box 3528
Littleton, CO 80161-3528

Toll-Free **1 (888) 209-0510**
Local (303) 224-0277
Fax (303) 224-0299

Web Site: **www.rmbarry.com**

E-mail: **info@rmbarry.com**

ISBN 0-9665924-3-3

Printed in the United States of America

Table of Contents

INTRODUCTION 1

Chapter 1 **THE MELALEUCA STORY** 3

Chapter 2 **THAT AMAZING TEA TREE OIL!** 19

Chapter 3 **GRAPE SEED EXTRACT** 39

Chapter 4 **GLUCOSAMINE the Arthritis Nutrient** . . . 45

Chapter 5 **IS YOUR HOME A HEALTHY HOME?** 49

Chapter 6 **HEALTHY BODY** 71
(see index for listing of conditions—pg. 82)

Chapter 7 **HEALTHY HOME** 159

Chapter 8 **HEALTHY PETS** 169

Chapter 9 **ALTERNATIVE USES** *(This is going to be a future chapter, but we need your help with it.)* 175

Appendix 1 **TEA TREE OIL RESEARCH** 176

Appendix 2 **DISINFECTANT PROPERTIES** 179

Appendix 3 **MELALEUCA OIL & HEALTHY SKIN** 180

Appendix 4 **48 KNOWN COMPOUNDS** 181

INDEX 182

ORDER INFORMATION 188

THE ULTIMATE
MELALEUCA
GUIDE

Introduction

We hope you enjoy this newly updated and greatly expanded version of the popular *Melaleuca Guide* book. Since 1995, the *Melaleuca Guide* has been the most authoritative and comprehensive resource for users of Melaleuca, Inc. products. Actually, earlier versions of the *Melaleuca Guide* go back as far as 1986, shortly after Melaleuca, Inc. was founded, and over 600,000 copies of different versions have been sold.

You will find that this latest version has been greatly expanded. In fact, this version has 60% more information than the previous edition. This is why we've decided to change the name of the book to *The Ultimate Melaleuca Guide*. I think you will find that the new name more accurately reflects the book's contents.

In this edition, we've added five new chapters as well as some additional information in the appendix section. We've also added several new health conditions which respond well to some of the newer Melaleuca products.

We have included a chapter called "The Melaleuca Story," mostly taken from our popular book *Built on Solid Principles: the Melaleuca Story* about the fascinating history of the company and the background and values of its founder and CEO, Frank VanderSloot.

Many of you have read our excellent booklet on tea tree oil by author Karen MacKenzie. We have now printed the entire contents of this fine booklet as a new chapter. You will also find a very complete listing of all relevant tea tree oil research as a new appendix in the back.

Many of you are also familiar with our *Is Your Home a Healthy Home?* booklet, having to do with the health effects of common household chemicals. You will find that the entire contents of this booklet are also included as a chapter. We've also added chapters on grape seed extract and glucosamine, taken from our other publications

We're confident you will find this newly updated and expanded *Melaleuca Guide* to be the most complete resource for Melaleuca users ever—and worthy of its new name, *The Ultimate Melaleuca Guide.*

CHAPTER ONE

1

The Melaleuca Story

by Richard M. Barry

Portions of this chapter have been taken from "Built On Solid Principles: the Melaleuca Story" by R.M. Barry. The book is a fascinating, in-depth portrayal of Frank VanderSloot, his mission, and how this former Idaho farm boy, once rated as lacking in leadership qualities, led Melaleuca, Inc. to phenomenal success in just a few short years. Informative, captivating, and truly inspirational, this fascinating portrait of a business founded on principles and integrity is a "must read" for anyone who wants to understand the company and the people who are drawn to it.

The story of Melaleuca, Inc. as we know it today actually began about fifteen years ago when a gifted American businessman had the insight to recognize the vast potential possessed by the unique substance we now call melaleuca oil, and the foresight to evolve a business strategy based on its therapeutic properties. That man is, of course, Frank VanderSloot, founder of Melaleuca, Inc.

The early days of the original company, Oil of Melaleuca, Inc. were beset with difficulty. At the time, Frank VanderSloot seemed an unlikely candidate for such a venture. He was already a successful man. His personal abilities had enabled him to rise above his simple origins in rural Idaho to become Regional Vice President of Cox Communications, Inc.

Initially, he was called into Oil of Melaleuca, Inc. by the Ball brothers who wanted a man of his prestige and prowess at the helm. They finally managed to convince Frank of the vast, untapped potential of this wonderful substance from Australia. After some investigation, Frank was sold on the product, and decided to join the Balls in the business, which had already been operating for several months. He intended to help out the Ball brothers for eighteen months and pick up his bonus check to pay off his new house—end of story.

It didn't quite work out that way.

On his first day at work, VanderSloot heard the tape of a radio interview given by one of the Ball brothers. This tape was being sold as a marketing tool, and when he listened to it VanderSloot was astounded to hear, among other claims, that melaleuca oil was being touted as a cure for herpes and gonorrhea. VanderSloot immediately ordered the tape to be withdrawn, but it was too late. The very next day, he was informed that a representative of the FDA was waiting to see him in the reception area.

In his speech at the Melaleuca Caribbean Cruise of 1999, Frank describes the incident very wittily: At first Frank was not worried. He went into the reception area, leaned across the oak desk and offered his hand to the FDA officer. Frank says, "Have you ever extended your hand to someone to shake it and they didn't shake it? It's not a good feeling. And that's what happened. I reached my hand out and instead of extending his, he reached into his back pocket and pulled out a wallet. A big, black wallet, and did what I know he'd done a hundred times before. He did a little flip with it. He flipped it open and it went 'thud!' right on that oak countertop and I was staring at the ugliest badge I have ever seen in my life. It said 'FDA'—and some other things on it—United States Government. He said: 'I'm Ed Edmunsen and I'm here to close your doors if you don't cease this illegal and unethical advertising.'"

With a gulp, Frank ushered the man into his office to be told in no uncertain terms he would not be allowed to operate while making such claims.

"I said, 'Hey, well you'll be happy to know, sir, today's my second day on the job and yesterday, my first day, I took that tape off the market. We're not selling it anymore. And besides, the guy that you're after is in Australia.'"

Frank later consulted an FDA expert to find that none of the literature could be used to promote Melaleuca. Whether the claims were true or not, in strict FDA terms, legally they could not be advertised.

Everything that could go wrong in a business did, though it was through no fault of Frank or the Ball brothers. Not only did the FDA totally clamp down on any advertising claims for the product, but the company's business plan floundered mainly because it was saddled with weaknesses inherited from an MLM-type structure.

The death knell was sounded with some more bad news. Frank had initially been attracted away from his secure job by the exciting potential of the oil itself. A partner in the business, an Australian plantation owner, had promised a world monopoly on the supply of high-grade oil. Given the enthusiasm that Frank had for the product after researching its benefits, the promise of a world monopoly had been a major clincher. It seemed too good to be true. And, in fact, it was. The Australian plantation owner's promises turned out to be false, and their world monopoly melted away.

Plagued with problems and unforeseen legal complications, VanderSloot and the Ball brothers made the inevitable decision to close the company.

Rather than see this as a failure, VanderSloot seized upon the demise of the original company as a starting point for an entirely new company. In doing so, he used the new company as the platform to launch an ideal so basically American that it seems innovative only because so many modern businesses have lost sight of it. Namely, that the Free Enterprise system does not have to be exploitative to succeed. To initiate his strategy, one of the first things VanderSloot did was to formulate a Mission Statement—*"Enhancing the Lives of Those We Touch by Helping People Reach Their Goals."*

From the beginning, Frank VanderSloot was adamant that the 'new' Melaleuca should help people to reach their goals in such a way that no one should get hurt, either in the business or by the business. This credo, coupled with his insistence on diligent legal and scientific research, led to the impeccable Melaleuca product line—"quality products made from natural substances supported by intensive research."

Perhaps the key to the heart of Melaleuca lies in VanderSloot's determination to "build a business to last a lifetime." Frank was a shrewd businessman and experience had taught him that continued growth needs two essential resources: product and personnel.

In the case of Melaleuca, where the Marketing Executives are drawn from people with homes and families—and full-time jobs—the only factor which will attract people and keep them is belief. It is impossible to foster this in people unless the products are the best and the morals of the company are beyond reproach.

Wary of the pitfalls of inventory loading and the multitude of traps in the MLM structure, VanderSloot evolved his now-famous system of Consumer Direct Marketing. Quite simply, it meant that any average person could gradually work towards financial independence, risk-free, without quitting his or her day job, spending vast amounts on products, or working countless hours processing customer orders on a monthly basis.

Listening to Frank VanderSloot's Melaleuca speeches over the years, it is possible to see how much his own personality has grown along with the company—a classic case of a man growing to fulfill the role he's defined for himself by sharing his heart-felt values. Though a fuller analysis of the man and his novel business methods are beyond the scope of this chapter, they are, in fact, covered in depth in a fascinating book *Built On Solid Principles: The Melaleuca Story.*

Frank's accomplishments are many. Not only does he serve on the Board of Directors of the prestigious United States Chamber of Commerce, but Idaho State University named him Business Leader of the Year, to mention but a few. Typically, VanderSloot shrugs off the glory of such successes, saying, "There were many people besides myself who contributed to Melaleuca's success."

Nevertheless, inadvertently, Frank tapped into something that is the model for new millennium business success as touted by America's top economic experts.

Charles Handy, "the philosopher for the world of business and management", foresaw in his book, The Age of Unreason, the collapse of the 45-year job and the paternalistic company which is taking place around us now. His blueprint for success in the next century provides a radical break with the 'take-no-prisoners' attitudes of 1990's business practice. Handy says: "The old-fashioned models of corporate control and contracts of employment are meaningless. Organizations have to be based on trust."

Similarly, Peter Drucker, one of the most perceptive observers of the American business scene stated: "The kind of organization [that will succeed] will be built around family and regional ties that, unlike American business, are personal rather than impersonal."

The fact is Frank VanderSloot must have gotten something right—the growth of Melaleuca has been staggering. In comparison with other product-based companies, there are no unseen pitfalls, no 'trickle-downs' from upper Executives making a fortune at the expense of those lower down the scale. The system works for everybody. Melaleuca's Marketing Executives have become a market force to reckon with and, as their scope and power have grown in keeping with the demands of the market, so has Melaleuca.

Despite these changes, the basic principles of Melaleuca have remained untouched. Time itself has shown that it is these very principles that have enabled Melaleuca to flourish at an amazing rate when traditional companies are going under. That these principles are touted by experts as "cutting-edge" may give rise to a chuckle. Melaleuca's principles were not formulated in an oak-paneled room in Princeton or Harvard. They are simply the down-home values Frank acquired from his hard-working Idaho father. It is these simple truths that empowered Melaleuca to rise above the shaky start of Oil of Melaleuca, Inc. and chart a path through the shark-infested waters of the 90's business world into the bright future of the next century.

It also attests to something that Frank VanderSloot believes we all possess: the ability to affect the lives of others in a positive way. He says: "We don't have to do great, newsworthy things to have a great influence on this world. We only need to live a life others can follow. It is impossible to measure the impact that one life can have on thousands of others."

VanderSloot calls this principle ...

THE POWER OF ONE

The success of Melaleuca is living proof of this principle for, in VanderSloot's case, his main influence—an influence that is prevalent everywhere in the 'Melaleuca philosophy'—came from his father.

Peter Francis VanderSloot is typical of the millions of "quiet Americans" who formed the backbone of America in the 1950s and, in many ways, enabled it to rise to its status as the leader of the economic world. They did this simply by being who they are: simple, working folk who work. And how they work. With only a third-grade education, Peter VanderSloot labored up to sixty hours a week on the railways, sometimes away from home a week at a time. He spent his whole life just feeding his kids and providing a home and values that would serve them in the future.

There is in such people a quiet wisdom which is the way of those who tend animals, till the soil and wake each morning without complaint, ready for a day of toil. Frank imbibed this wisdom from his father wholesale—and is eternally grateful for it. He says: "If I had not had the influence of my father in my life... it's doubtful that Melaleuca would exist as it does today."

Life on a small farm is not easy. Rural Idaho in those days was very poor. Work was hard to come by and it was mostly just logging. Such environments breed common sense, and Mr. VanderSloot, Sr., instilled his values in Frank not by preaching sermons but by practical example. For example, when he wanted Frank to have the education he had missed himself, he gave Frank a milk cow! Frank would milk that cow morning and night. He'd churn up the milk with a hand paddle and, making sure to keep his brother away from the final product, Frank would sell the cream for a few dollars at the market. Amazingly, Frank used this money to finance his college education. And, in keeping with the hard lesson learned, he actually paid for his own college expenses by living in and watching over a Laundromat.

It was quite an eye-opener for Frank seeing people at college with new clothes when all his were bought at the Salvation Army thrift store, but he was never jealous. In fact, it reinforced his first lessons: keep out of debt, work hard and, as he never heard his father tell a lie, always be honest.

For those approaching the Melaleuca organization for the first time or even those within it, it is important to understand VanderSloot's assertion that he is "not especially gifted." In his early years, he actually hated standing up in front of people and failed a leadership-attitude test because of his shyness. But through the example of his father and other key figures in his life, he came to realize the importance of self-esteem and the impact that the right kind of influence can have on the future of a so-called "average" person.

After the demise of Oil of Melaleuca, Inc., VanderSloot had to work late into the night to salvage a viable business from its shipwreck. He was not simply struggling with facts and figures. Rather, he was determined to develop a business that was built on the solid foundation of his home values. Also, it had to be a business that was readily available to not just a gifted few but to anyone with the desire and determination to succeed.

In picturing Frank at this stage, it should be remembered that when he began with Oil of Melaleuca, Inc., he was already a very successful businessman. As Regional Vice President of Cox Communications, Inc., a Fortune 500 company, he'd served his time in the 'war trenches' of modern business and had come out tops. The fact is, once the initial shock of the Oil of Melaleuca, Inc. failure had settled, he realized that he now had the chance to start something new, something that had been hovering at the back of his mind for years.

He embarked on a quest for knowledge. He consulted marketing gurus, direct-sales experts and FDA attorneys. From them he took what he thought was the best and incorporated it into his own methodology. What he came up with was a risk-free plan with a low monthly production requirement well within the scope of any American household.

The plan was elegant in its structure, economically sound—and innovative. VanderSloot was no longer in pursuit of a dream but possessed of a viable strategy to facilitate it. It was to become no less than the 'Melaleuca Way'.

THE MELALEUCA WAY

"Give a man a fish; it feeds him for a day. Teach him how to fish and he can feed himself for a lifetime." VanderSloot's idea was not to give away opportunity but to empower people to make their own. And from the well of this simple philosophy have sprung many statements and slogans which are at the heart of the Melaleuca experience:

- "No one must get hurt from what we do."
- "The magic is in helping others reach their goals and not in trying to reach our own goals."
- "No amount of wealth will bring true happiness if it is gained unethically."
- "We are not a multi-level company... Multi-level marketing has been used to con [people] into money-making schemes. We have never done that."
- "We don't have a right to be here unless we are marketing the best products for the best prices at the best value of anybody in this nation."
- "Don't quit your job."
- "We're telling about Melaleuca, not selling it."
- "The marketing and delivery of exceptional products at reasonable prices has been the key to our success."

Hundreds of thousands of people are now taking advantage of the opportunity to compete against the huge conglomerates. Marketing

Executives are pulling customers away from these giants in tens of thousands by using Melaleuca's unique Marketing Plan.

However, when VanderSloot hears his Executives enthusing about his "wonderful Marketing Plan," he gives them a few home-truths. "I feel that sometimes there's a tendency for people to perceive that it's the Marketing Plan that brings us our success. It is not so." His conviction is deep on this matter. "Without having the best products that money can buy, we don't really have an excuse to be here."

THE BEST OF SCIENCE & NATURE

It is for this reason that he was determined that, in the future, Melaleuca would use only those products that were the very best in nature, as supported and guided by scientific research. VanderSloot sought tirelessly to form relationships with pharmacists, nutritional experts, allopathic and homeopathic doctors, herbal experts, and scientists from all fields. His aim was to sort out the product wheat from product chaff.

As an illustration of how VanderSloot spent his time during this period, here's an example of one of his contacts. Frank located a doctor who was something of an expert on tea tree oil. For more than ten years, this man had been using the oil in his practice to treat a wide variety of complaints. Frank spent the entire day with the doctor, extracting every scrap of information he could about the uses of tea tree oil and the various mixtures used to treat different complaints. They must have been mutually impressed with each other because when Frank established Melaleuca, Inc., the man became a loyal customer. So much so that in 1986 the doctor published his first book about Melaleuca products. Then, in 1995, the doctor greatly expanded his book and called it the *Melaleuca Guide*. It is said that the test of time is the true judge of all things. If so, his books have passed with flying colors, since over 600,000 copies have been sold. In fact, a historical footnote is that this worthy doctor has since moved on to other things. However, the book in your hand at the moment, *The Ultimate Melaleuca Guide,* is a new and radically-revised book, but is still based on all the tried and tested product knowledge from the original *Melaleuca Guide.*

THE PIONEER PRODUCT: MELALEUCA OIL

To create the exceptional product line he needed for the new company, VanderSloot had to have a dependable supply of high-grade melaleuca oil. He went to great lengths to secure a crop which could propagate a superior tree line. No two strains of the *Melaleuca alternifolia* tree provided the same quality of oil. His investigations took him to Australia. The best stands of *Melaleuca alternifolia* trees are in an area called the Bungawalbyn Reserve™. The Bungawalbyn varieties produce genetically-superior trees that give the highest quality oil. The properties of the tree were so highly thought of by the local Aborigines that the very word *Bungawalbyn* means 'healing ground'. Thus, VanderSloot was able to secure exclusive rights to oil harvested from natural stands; these Bungawalbyn trees had never been treated with herbicides or pesticides.

Under Melaleuca's incentive, the growers sought out more robust and higher-yield trees, took seedlings from them, and from this superior line began establishing plantations of trees. The enthusiastic participation of the Australian growers was ensured by Melaleuca who supported them through years of poor yields, and the growers responded with a greater diligence in producing the highest-quality yield possible.

As research on melaleuca oil progressed, it became obvious that its medicinal properties were directly proportional to its quality of oil. Higher grades of the oil have greater levels of the therapeutic agent Terpinen 4-ol and less of Cineole, which can be irritating to sensitive skin.

Other companies were selling substandard grades of the oil as "pure oil of *Melaleuca alternifolia*." Some of these oils have very little, if any, medicinal value. VanderSloot wanted to make sure that Melaleuca sold only the highest-quality oil available, and that customers could clearly see what grade they were getting. He decided to place the grade designation right on the label, and hence the name "*T36-C7*" for the standard high-grade oil, and "*T40-C5*" for the ultra-rare grade oil. These pure oils have been shown to be superlative treatments for stings, burns, skin rashes and a host of topical applications. Because the higher grade of the oil comes from trees with rare genetics and the supply is limited, it is more expensive.

Melaleuca recently raised the standards for both grades of their oil to "*T36-C5*" and "*T40-C3*," which demonstrates a commitment to making the very best oil available as growing and harvesting techniques continue to improve. The standard high-grade oil is used in a wide range of Melaleuca products, most notably in skin care, hair care, dental care, and medicine chest products.

Even though reputable organizations the world over have validated melaleuca oil's effectiveness and safety, VanderSloot is always cautious about its claims. By 1996, over six million bottles of the oil had been sold. Nevertheless, when describing its uses, Frank insisted on erring on the conservative side, saying, "It's clear that melaleuca oil has some very unique and unusual properties. Many people have experimented and reported very favorable results on conditions such as cold sores, canker sores, candida, chicken pox, herpes, thrush, etc. Several studies have been done on some of these conditions that appear quite promising. But more research needs to be done to verify its efficacy before being able to make legitimate claims in regard to these conditions."

The book is not yet closed on melaleuca oil. In some ways, it is still a mystery and, as of yet, not all of its properties are fully understood. New research is expanding its possibilities every day. One thing is certain—as new uses are discovered for this wonderful substance, Melaleuca will ensure that any potential benefit is passed on to customers.

BEYOND MELALEUCA OIL

Nearly 30% of Melaleuca's revenues go into product quality. Compared to this, traditional manufacturers only spend about 10% for the same purpose. By pouring revenue back into product development, Melaleuca has been able to provide an ever-widening range of new products, many of which are not based on melaleuca oil at all.

Melaleuca's research and development team continually searches for natural ingredients with known restorative or curative powers. Having found such an ingredient, Melaleuca will either closely examine any former research on it, or they will initiate fresh research. As a result of such investigations, Melaleuca now distributes a line of products which use ingredients that go far beyond the original flagship product, *Melaleuca oil*. Nowadays, many of the products are not based on the oil at all but on other natural botanicals—plants and herbs whose health-promoting properties have been known for years and whose viability has been established by further testing. These include household products that are safe to both the health of the user and that of the environment, and a wide range of personal care and cosmetic products.

Americans are slowly becoming aware that protecting our health and the environment is not just the province of the fanatical few. The gap between the violation of nature's delicate balance and its rebound effect on humanity is growing narrower every year. Melaleuca's household and personal care products offer a solution where the giant corporations have simply turned a blind eye. This has created a competitive edge for the company as it attracts more and more people who realize they can now exercise personal and environmental responsibility without sacrificing effectiveness.

UNLOCKING NATURE'S SECRETS WITH SCIENCE

As Melaleuca expanded, there seems to be a peculiar sense of appropriateness in the direction taken. Following its establishment of safe household and personal care products, Melaleuca's move into the area of nutrition and personal health aids seemed a natural step. "We have found that mother nature has provided a natural solution for almost every health problem that confronts us. Our task is to use science as the key to unlock the secrets that nature has to offer," states VanderSloot.

As Melaleuca R&D uncovers fresh developments in natural health, the flexibility of their infrastructure facilitates their ability to investigate and incorporate such developments into an enhanced product line. This is accomplished on a time scale which would be impossible for the gigantic corporations. Not only does this put Melaleuca on the cutting edge, but the speed at which it takes place does not compromise safety or quality.

FRUCTOSE COMPOUNDING

Given some of the negative factors of modern life—stress, pollution, over-processed foods—it is even more essential that our body receive an adequate supply of vitamins and especially minerals. A healthy diet which includes the recommended intake of fruits and vegetables does not always provide the necessary nutrition. If the minerals are not in the soil, they won't be reproduced in the food. Thus, the degeneration of soil quality and the practice of over-processing food has given rise to a peculiar phenomenon—people who overeat and are still malnourished.

Furthermore, nutritional research has also shown that even when there is an adequate mineral supply within certain foods, it doesn't necessarily mean that the body will receive the full benefit. This anomaly came to the attention of nutritionists in Egypt, Libya, and Iran in the 70's, where children were suffering from horrible symptoms of zinc deficiency—severe growth retardation and dwarfism—even though the local foods contained an adequate supply of zinc.

The explanation is that the zinc attaches itself to certain acids in the food and is passed right through the body as "waste," without even getting to the cells. This happens, though to a lesser degree, with the minerals in our diets as well. The problem is solved by using an innovative process which binds a mineral to fructose, a substance found in fruit which is very readily absorbed by the cells. By using this "fruit sugar" messenger to carry the minerals piggy-back style, the mineral is passed through to the tissues and its full benefits can be utilized by the body.

This patented process called "fructose compounding" is exclusive to Melaleuca. No one else has this cutting-edge technology, which is one of the features of Melaleuca's *Vitality Pak,* a health product delivered to the customer's door in the shape of fifty-five vitamins and fructose-compounded minerals.

THE CASE OF BOBBI MCCAUGHEY

Melaleuca's emphasis on using only those quality products which have been validated and well researched has had some interesting repercussions in the community at large. Not the least of these is the case of Bobbi McCaughey, the Iowa woman whose claim to fame is the delivery of seven living children at one birth.

To fully appreciate the magnitude of this feat, it has to be remembered that formerly in cases of multiple births, all or some of the children died. In fact in two previous cases of septuplet births, all the babies died.

When Bobbi had recovered from the news that she was pregnant seven times over (if, indeed, she ever will recover!), the primary concern was her physical robustness. Could she withstand the severe assault of this incredible event?

Her pastor's wife, Ginny Brown, is a Melaleuca Marketing Executive. Ginny suggested that Bobbi use *The Vitality Pak*. Of course, Bobbi had to have her doctors look over the specifications of *The Vitality Pak*. They examined the ingredients closely before approving them. Bobbi embarked upon a regimen of three *Mel-Vita* and *Mela-Cal* tablets, and three *ProVex-Plus* capsules daily. The most distinctive advantage of *The Vitality Pak* is the high absorption of minerals due to Melaleuca's patented fructose-compounding process.

Bobbi says, "We thought it would be a great help during the pregnancy and that it would be much more usable—as far as being absorbed by my body—than a regular prenatal vitamin would be."

A pregnant woman has very special nutritional needs. For instance, Bobbi was supposed to eat 4,000 calories a day, but she could not eat that much. "I needed to eat something every forty minutes and I just couldn't."

Zinc and calcium are especially needed, even during a normal pregnancy. In this case, the situation was even more extreme—Bobbi was carrying seven babies. So it was absolutely essential that she had the right nutrition. But, for the first five months of the pregnancy, she was so sick she could hardly eat at all. Once she got to the hospital she was able to eat a little bit more, but she says, "But then I had hospital food, so I didn't want to eat any more! So it was good to have something that was really able to boost the vitamins and minerals I didn't get from the food."

The circumstances of a pregnancy seven times over needed very special precautions. Bobbi was told by her doctors to stay in bed for the last five months of the pregnancy. This immediately introduced other possible problems—blood clotting in the legs, reduced muscle tone, and loss of bone mass. Also, a common aspect of multiple pregnancies is that blood pressure can rapidly escalate to abnormal proportions. The doctors who had examined the ingredients of *The Vitality Pak* told Bobbi to take three *Mela-Cal* and three *Mel-Vita* tablets every day, and she never had any problems with blood pressure.

Ginny, knowing that it might be difficult for the McCaughey's to pay for the vitamins in such quantities, called Tish Poling at Melaleuca, and Tish discreetly arranged that the McCaughey's would get everything they needed from Melaleuca without any intrusive publicity.

When Bobbi was asked how she felt during this period, she replied, "I felt really good. It wasn't until probably the last week and a half that I really felt terrible. By that time, the contractions had started and I was on other medications to stop them."

Of course, Frank VanderSloot was proud that Melaleuca's vitamins and minerals had been used in such a medically-sensitive situation. He said, "We're really pleased that the McCaugheys decided to use our vitamins, and that the result has been so great. Our hopes and prayers are with them as they prepare for the wonderful experiences ahead."

Well, the results have become worldwide news. Bobbi did deliver her seven bouncing bundles of joy—the first woman in known history to do so. Of course, Bobbi's major feat attracted worldwide attention. One day, when Bobbi was back in the hospital post-delivery, the phone rang. Ken McCaughey picked up the phone. A voice said, "Mr. McCaughey, you have a phone call from the President of the United States."

The McCaugheys were astonished. The President had phoned to offer his personal congratulations. Bobbi's marathon feat had even caught the imagination of the President of the United States!

Naturally, the credit should go to Bobbi and her team of doctors. Still, there is no doubt that Melaleuca's policy of credible testing and high-quality product meant that *The Vitality Pak* was well up to their standards.

A comic side-light to the Bobbi McCaughey case took place during one of Frank VanderSloot's talks. While addressing a roomful of people, Frank mentioned that Bobbi had been taking *The Vitality Pak*.

"All of a sudden," Frank said, "from the back of the room, a woman screamed, 'OH MY GOSH!!' It seems she was a new customer and she'd just started taking *The Vitality Pak* herself. She was concerned that somehow that was what caused the seven babies!"

Partly because of Bobbi McCaughey's experience with *The Vitality Pak*, Melaleuca has now introduced *The Vitality Pak Prenatal*. This new formulation is specifically designed for the nutritional needs of a woman during her pregnancy.

THE *ACCESS BAR*

As we move into the first century of the new millennium, the greatest change in health care is the trend towards prevention rather than cure. In particular, lifestyle has been designated as a major causal factor in disease.

Exercise is a key element in a healthy lifestyle. Obesity is a major concern, and lack of exercise is a main contributor to strokes and heart attacks. The *Access Bar* was developed specially to ensure that the maximum possible benefits were obtained from exercise.

Through Melaleuca's practice of networking with cutting-edge doctors, they became aware of Dr. Lawrence Wang's studies into fat metabolism. Dr. Wang, Ph.D., is the Professor of Animal and Human Physiology at the University of Alberta, Edmonton, Canada, and a member of the prestigious Royal Society of Canada.

His research into fat metabolism led him to a substance called adenosine which exerts a blocking effect on the burning of stored fat during exercise. Adenosine, a by-product of activity, leads to the familiar sensation in fatigued muscles, expressed in the old exercise slogan as "feel the burn." It is adenosine which is indirectly responsible for that burning sensation and muscle soreness after exercise. Normally, exercise burns off glucose, not fat, but by utilizing a natural substance which inhibits the effect of the adenosine, Wang was able to increase the direct burning of fat, not glucose, during exercise.

This led to the *Access Fat-Conversion Activity Bar,* a product made from natural substances which has become a mainstay for both athletes and casual exercisers alike. Taken approximately fifteen minutes before exercise, the bar ensures that the body will burn less glucose and more fat. Fatigue and soreness are minimized and exercise can continue for longer periods. This simple, safe exercise bar ensures that maximum benefits can be attained during any exercise routine.

THE EVOLUTION OF PROVEX CV™

Melaleuca's interest in formidable health issues did not stop with obesity. In 1995, Melaleuca announced that they were committed to becoming a world leader in research and development into a group of substances known as flavonoids. This was in direct response to the enormous medical problem of heart disease and the related medical and lifestyle factors associated with it.

The results have been quite amazing. VanderSloot remarked: "We never dreamed that when we said we would become a world leader, we would actually become the world leader in the development of products to reduce the risk of heart disease."

Melaleuca's interest in flavonoids had been aroused by a peculiar phenomenon known as the French Paradox which came to the attention of the public in 1990. The way in which the story develops is a prime example of Melaleuca's product development methodology.

Apparently, the French consume 2.8 times the amount of lard as Americans and 3.8 times as much butter. The French are also a nation of very heavy smokers. Yet, despite the fact that they have higher blood cholesterol levels and higher blood pressure readings than Americans, the French have only one-third the rate of heart attacks.

Subsequent research led scientists to attribute this odd paradox to the French's habitual consumption of red wine with meals. This led to further studies into the constituents of red wine, aimed at pinpointing the connection between the wine and their lowered incidence of heart attacks. Over the years, many such experiments gradually eliminated different factors until, finally, something concrete was established. It seems the lowered incidence of heart attacks in the French was due to a substance in grape skins and seeds known as flavonoids. Flavonoids are present in red wine and purple grape juice.

The basic causes of heart attacks had already been well established by earlier researchers. It stems from two factors—the buildup of "oxidized" cholesterol on artery walls, which causes the artery to become restricted, and the "stickiness" of blood platelets which may cause a blockage in the restricted artery.

The buildup of "bad" cholesterol has been shown to be minimized by antioxidants such as Vitamin E. Also, as early as 1974 it was demonstrated that aspirin can reduce artery blockage by inhibiting platelet clotting.

This simplified explanation indicates that any attempt to reduce heart attacks has to be a two-fold attack—one, to produce an antioxidant that reduces the oxidation of "bad" cholesterol; and two, to reduce blood platelet "stickiness" in a similar manner to the action of aspirin.

Aspirin has one major drawback. Most heart attacks are induced through stress, and it was found that aspirin's effect is minimized in the presence of adrenaline, which is released during stress—the "Catch 22" of using aspirin for this purpose.

Melaleuca, in responding to the challenge of this new area, formed an alliance with Dr. John Folts, the man who had conducted the original research into the beneficial effects of aspirin. Folts had already spent several years researching the effects of flavonoids on platelet stickiness. He believed that flavonoids were the key to the 'French paradox'. Folts says, "Focusing on flavonoid supplements was the next logical step. Everyone has been asking when they'll be able to get the same benefits [of red wine] from a pill."

Melaleuca's goal was to develop a flavonoid-based dietary supplement that would be effective at preventing heart disease. Initial research revealed that flavonoids extracted from plants are not absorbed completely by the body. At first this was very disappointing news.

Other manufacturers of flavonoid supplements were touting them as being effective against heart disease based on tests which were done in test tubes only. Melaleuca's research had been done in living subjects and clearly showed that the claims made by the other manufacturers were greatly exaggerated.

The researchers set out to solve the problem of absorption so the benefits of the flavonoids could be utilized by the body. After almost two years they discovered that a particular mixture of flavonoid extracts combined with a special blend of enzymes greatly increased the absorption of the flavonoids. This was the breakthrough they had been looking for. This led to the development of the first flavonoid-based supplement which has been proven (in living subjects) to be effective in curbing the two primary causes of heart disease.

"WHEN THE TRUTH IS ALMOST TOO GOOD TO BE TRUE"

This was the title of Frank VanderSloot's September 1997 President's Message, which was a direct response to the results of Dr. Folts' research. These results, to put it mildly, were overwhelming. A ripple of excitement fluttered through the Melaleuca world as the breakthrough product, known as *ProVexCV*, was made available to Melaleuca Marketing Executives at the 1997 Convention.

Frank VanderSloot, in accordance with long-established Melaleuca principles, asked for restraint. He urged his Marketing Executives to refrain from any publicity until Dr. Folts and his researchers could publish their findings in appropriate medical journals.

Melaleuca's success with *ProVexCV* is not a lucky accident. Melaleuca is ever sifting through the enormous number of natural remedies to all kinds of illnesses. The larger corporations simply will not take time to investigate natural remedies. One reason for this is they cannot be patented. And smaller companies simply don't have the funds to pursue the kind of research that led to *ProVexCV*. So Melaleuca has carved out a huge niche for itself in the marketplace as the leading manufacturer of beneficial natural products.

In his February 1997 address, Frank VanderSloot illustrated the importance of R&D: "If any company, large or small, comes out with a great product, rather than competing with it, we'll incorporate it into our own product line—and we will challenge our own scientists to improve on it. We did exactly that with *ProVex*—instead of becoming a competitor or follower in that industry, we found a better way, and we became the leader."

Melaleuca, Inc.'s astute methods of uncompromising testing have borne fruit in more ways than one. In the words of Frank VanderSloot, "As our ongoing research continues to uncover more of nature's secrets, we promise to keep you informed. We believe this is a never-ending story, but the first chapter is now complete ... Stay tuned for more information."

Well, more information did come and this time it raised a ripple of excitement not just amongst Melaleuca Executives but the world.

The Press has always been intrigued by the idea of the French Paradox—the idea that drinking alcohol could actually promote health is something of a teaser. Unfortunately, this was always its weak point medically.

Then, in November 1998, Dr. Folts delivered a presentation to the American Dietetic Association. In the context of numerous other presentations, this was the one that attracted the attention of the Press.

Folts had experimented with a supplement consisting of carefully researched amounts of grape seed, grape skin, Gingko biloba, bilberries and a specific flavonoid called quercetin. Folts found that his test subjects showed a "significant and encouraging" reduction in the contributing factors responsible for heart disease.

This was the news that sent the Press racing for the door. The news was circulated very rapidly via Associated Press, Reuters, and numerous other agencies. Over 100 articles were generated in different newspapers around the nation and on numerous television news programs. Here was absolute verification that a non-alcoholic substance in pill form could be effective against heart disease.

Folts' talk was a major breakthrough. But for Melaleuca, it was, in some sense, old hat. For, of course, the supplement Folts tested was none other than *ProVexCV*.

Earlier that year, VanderSloot had said, "We have also learned some exciting things about the most effective way to extract the nutrients from grape seeds and grape skins ... We have learned exactly how to do it and we are not telling anyone else. And much of what we know is now protected by patent."

A patent? Yes. Melaleuca, Inc. had the foresight to contract with the only manufacturer who knew the special process needed to obtain the maximum result from the grapes. Melaleuca even arranged with the manufacturer to have a special factory built. Melaleuca's contract ensures that they, and only they, are eligible to receive this special extract for the next twenty years.

It is ironic that fifteen years earlier Frank VanderSloot had taken over the reins of a new company based on the promise of another monopoly—the world monopoly of melaleuca oil. Sadly, it turned out to be too good to be true. Now, fifteen years later, Melaleuca, Inc. stands on the threshold of an incredible medical coup. And this time, the monopoly is signed, sealed, and water-tight.

As the new millennium dawns and Melaleuca trembles on the brink of a solution to America's Number One health problem, the future is looking brighter than Frank VanderSloot could ever have dreamed. With an air of barely-concealed excitement, he states:

"I do not know of any company, regardless of size, let alone a Direct Marketing company, that has had the opportunity to take a product of this magnitude to market. A product that is so far advanced beyond anything else in the marketplace ...! It's wonderful to be in a position where the truth is almost too good to be true. Thank goodness it *is* true. I cannot imagine a better situation for us to be in."

Indeed.

CHAPTER TWO

2

That Amazing Tea Tree Oil!

ABOUT THE AUTHOR

Karen MacKenzie began her investigation into Tea Tree oil in 1989 while working as a researcher for an essential oil company. During this time, she began to develop a strong interest in alternative medicine and nutrition. When, in 1991, she developed an allergy to chemicals in many personal care products and make-up, she was forced to search for chemical-free alternatives. Unfortunately, there were very few alternatives available back then. Her quest led her to begin using Tea Tree oil in a variety of ways with spectacular results, and her allergy eventually subsided.

She began writing about Tea Tree oil to share her experiences with others. In 1996, she founded the Tea Tree Oil Information Service in Great Britain to help spread the word and to assist medical professionals as well as the general public in using this valuable natural gift.

INTRODUCTION

When I initially heard about Tea Tree oil, I could not believe it. It was too good to be true. Why had we not heard about it before? The truth is we had, but then we had chosen to ignore it!

I have traced Tea Tree oil back to its roots in Aboriginal Australia, through its popularity during the Second World War, right up to the present day world-wide acclaim. I have read the research papers, used it for first aid applications, treated my pets, and even cleaned many household accessories and furnishings with it.

I am constantly amazed by its versatility and effectiveness. I would never have believed that an essential oil from one plant could lend itself so successfully to so many different applications. No one but God, through nature, could have created such a valuable broad-spectrum substance, and that is the beauty of Tea Tree oil—it is totally natural.

I wrote this in an effort to bring Tea Tree oil to your attention, so you, like I, could read about its history, study the research work, utilize its many properties, and make up your own mind about nature's potent gift. After all, Tea Tree oil was created for each and every one of us.

PREFACE

Every week we see the same headlines in the newspapers "Head Lice Shampoo Cancer Scare" ... "The Age of the Superbug is Here" ... "Household Chemicals and Pollution Linked to Cancer" ... "Acne Treatment Damages Skin Cells" ... and so on.

We are now just beginning to wake up to the fact that the synthetic chemical cocktails we encounter during the course of a lifetime—hairsprays, cosmetics, deodorants, polishes, detergents, toothpastes, perfumes, aftershaves, first aid treatments, medicines, air fresheners, etc.—are systematically weakening our bodies. It is undeniable that our health is beginning to suffer. Where will it all end?

Germs, bacteria, and other parasites are evolving to beat their chemical killers. The "superbugs," including MRSA (Golden staph), thrive. Mystery illnesses are on the increase. Do we then try to make stronger chemicals? You bet we do!

Are we not forgetting one simple, fundamental fact? Bacteria is a basic, one-celled form of life, and these chemicals are harmful to all life—including our own!! When we use harsh chemicals against bacteria we can also unbalance and even destroy our own body cells, too.

I am not denying that synthetic medicine was, and is, a great gift. But it is its indiscriminate use, in addition to all other synthetics and chemicals, that is causing the problem. Over fifty years ago society started to turn its back on nature, and the chemical industry took center stage. We seemed to forget that we were part of nature and that to turn against it, we would be turning against ourselves. It is only now that we are beginning to pay the price.

Now, wouldn't it be marvelous if we could find a safe, non-toxic, non-irritating substance that would play a role in replacing many of the strong chemicals in our cupboards? Well, we have!

Here is a product that is made by nature, for nature. It is a completely natural, topical, clinically proven anti-bacterial and anti-fungal substance. It has anti-inflammatory, immune system strengthening, pain killing, and wound healing qualities. It also exhibits anti-viral, expectorant, and balsamic characteristics.

All this, and it can be used as a powerful antiseptic, parasiticide and insecticide. AND it's also kind to our skin cells. The pure Tea Tree oil of the *Melaleuca alternifolia,* works with the body, not against it. Research shows it has rapid results against the new "20th Century Superbugs" including MRSA.

I still find it ironic that if man had made such a synthetic substance and had spent millions of dollars on the development program, it would have been hailed as the wonder of the century. Everyone would have known about it, and everyone would be utilizing its many properties. But because Tea Tree oil is found in nature, it is viewed with suspicion.

The sooner we all once again wholeheartedly embrace a more natural approach in both medicine and in industry, the sooner we will begin to stem the tide of the so called "superbugs" and "mystery illnesses."

THE TEA TREE OIL STORY

To trace the history of the "healing Tea Trees" we have to start on the North Eastern coastal region of New South Wales, Australia—the only place in the world where the *Melaleuca alternifolia* tree yields the "real" Tea Tree oil.

We then have to travel back centuries, long before Australia was "discovered," and long before scientific evidence began, to a time when Australia belonged to its native inhabitants, the Aborigines. In particular, the Bundjalong Aborigines inhabited the wetlands around the Bungawalbyn Creek and, according to legend, were well aware of the medicinal qualities of their many "healing trees." Although not documented, it is widely understood that they treated various wounds and skin infections with an early form of poultice made from crushed leaves and warm mud from along the banks of the creek. The poultice was excellent for drawing out infection and healing the skin.

These Aborigines also used the healing waters of the pools in the area which were surrounded by the trees. Falling leaves and twigs leached their "magical" healing liquid into the water, turning it a deep yellowish color. The Aborigines bathed and washed in this natural healing "spa" to treat any number of conditions from sore muscles to serious diseases. Maybe this is why they named the area "Bungawalbyn" in the first place. The name means "healing ground."

The "healing trees" did not become commonly known as "Tea Trees" until around 1770 when Captain Cook, along with a botanist named Joseph Banks and the crew of The Endeavour, used the leaves with their distinctive aroma to brew a spicy and refreshing "tea." It is most unfortunate that they did not "discover" and publish the unique healing qualities of the "Tea Trees." But according to the account of that time, they drank the essence in varying concoctions, even alcoholic beverages such as a "Tea Tree beer."

Thus the name "Tea Tree" became popular, especially with the first "white" settlers who colonized the low-lying areas around the Clarence and Richmond Rivers. From the 1790's on, they watched and learned from the Aborigines how to use the leaves and waters in various inhalations, poultices, and rubbing mediums. Because these first settlers rarely had medical or botanical backgrounds, there was no real "scientific" evidence recording the healing qualities of the Tea Trees. The European community was very skeptical of these "anecdotal stories." It could not have helped that the Aborigines were often thought of as primitives from an uncivilized world. In the words of the settlers, "They didn't want to work or better themselves ... they were always disobedient and lazy." Thus the healing remedies, along with the Aboriginal way of life, were treated with contempt.

As new settlers arrived, they struggled to clear the harsh native vegetation to make way for settlements and dairy farms. They cursed every Tea Tree for its hardy and persistent hold on its own natural habitat. The Tea Trees tenaciously survived drought, fire, flood, and even frost, and resisted any attempt to destroy them. Fortunately for the rest of the world, the only way they could have been eradicated was by the physical removal of every part of the tree, including the extensive root system.

It is ironic that while the settlers battled to destroy the Tea Trees, they were only too willing to use the healing leaves for poultices and inhalations to stem infection and disease.

It is to our loss that the Tea Tree, although used as an effective "bush remedy" by subsequent generations of farmers, did not reach our attention until the early 1930's. It was not even mentioned in the *British Pharmaceutical Codex* until 1949, where it was listed as *"Oleum Melaleuca."* [1]

In Australia it was not until the early 1920's that Arthur de Ramon Penfold, FCS, Chief Chemist at the Museum of Applied Technology, Arts and Sciences in Sydney, extracted the oil of the Melaleuca alternifolia and announced that "yes indeed!" it did have antiseptic and anti-bacterial properties.[2] The accepted anti-bacterial agent at that time was carbolic acid (known as phenol). Imagine the stir it must have caused when it was determined that "an old Aboriginal remedy" was up to 13 times stronger! and was non-toxic and non-irritating—unlike carbolic acid! [3]

When the results were finally published in 1925, there was great enthusiasm among doctors of the time and "Penfold's discovery" was immediately put to the test.

In 1930 the *Medical Journal of Australia* published an article, "A New Australian Germicide," by Dr. E.M. Humphrey.[4] It stated "that what he found most encouraging was the way that the oil from the crushed leaves of the *Melaleuca alternifolia* dissolved pus and left wounds and surrounding areas clean." He tested and enthused about this great substance, highlighting Tea Tree oil as never before.

He noticed "that the germicidal action became more effective in the

1 "Oleum Melaleuca," *British Pharmaceutical Codex,* 597-598, 1949.
2 Penfold, A.R. and Grant, R. "The Germicidal Values of Some Australian Essential Oils and Their Pure Constituents," *Journal Proceedings of the Royal Society of NSW,* 59:3, 346-50, 1925.
3 This was determined by the Rideal-Walker co-efficient, a method used at that time to determine the germicidal properties of compounds.
4 Humphrey, E.M. "A New Australian Germicide," *Medical Journal of Australia,* I, 417-418, 1930.

presence of living tissue and organic matter, without any apparent damage to healthy cells." ...

He suggested "that it would be particularly good for applying to dirty wounds caused in street accidents." ...

He also found "most encouraging the results on nail infections. Particularly those infections that had resisted various treatments for months which now were cured in less than a week!" ...

"The pus solvent properties of Tea Tree oil made it an excellent application for the fungal nail disease paronychia, which if left untreated could result in the deformity and even eventual loss of the nail." ...

He urged the dental industry to "take seriously the antiseptic properties for infections of the gum and mouth." ...

He noted that "just two drops of Tea Tree oil in a tumbler of warm water made it a soothing and therapeutic gargle for sore throats in the early stages." ...

He wrote that "it would probably be effective for most of the infections of the naso-pharynx." ...

That it "was an immediate deodorizing medium on foul-smelling wounds and pus-filled abscesses." ...

And, "if it was added to hand soap it would make the soap up to sixty times more effective against Typhoid bacilli than the so-called 'disinfectant soaps' of the day." ...

He felt "that if an ointment could be made from the oil it would help to eradicate several parasitic skin diseases." ...

He concluded "that it was a rare occurrence because most effective germicides actually destroyed healthy living tissue along with the bacteria." ...

The Scientific and Medical worlds were intrigued. More research was funded and articles began appearing in additional publications such as the *Australian Journal of Pharmacy* [5] and the *Australian Journal of Dentistry.*[6] World-wide appetites were whetted. Articles were presented and published in the *Journal of the National Medical Association* (USA)[7] and the *British Medical Journal.*[8]

As the reputation of Tea Tree oil spread, there was a great deal of anecdotal evidence about its effectiveness in a wide range of topical applications, both medical and veterinary. From diabetic gangrene in man[9] to diseases of poultry and fish, it was recognized as a safe, effective, non-toxic, non-irritating, antiseptic disinfectant.[10]

---

5 Anon, "Tea Tree Oil," *Australian Journal of Pharmacy,* p274, 30th March 1930.
6 MacDonald, V. "The Rationale of Treatment," *Australian Journal of Dentistry,* 34, 281-285, 1930.
7 Anon, *Journal of the National Medical Association* (USA), 1930.
8 Anon, "Ti-trol Oil," *British Medical Journal,* 927, 1933.
8 Anon, "An Australian Antiseptic Oil," *British Medical Journal,* 966, 1933.
9 Halford, A.C.F. "Diabetic Gangrene," *Medical Journal of Australia,* 2, 121-122, 1936.
10 Penfold, A.R. and Morrison, F.R. "Some Notes on the Essential Oil of *Melaleuca alternifolia,*" *Australian Journal of Pharmacy,* 18, 274-5, 1937.

If Penfold was the "Founding Father," Humphrey was certainly the "Metaphorical Mother." His enthusiastic writings opened up a multitude of medical and practical uses for Tea Tree oil. Others have tried, tested, and approved of its healing properties, but thanks to Penfold and Humphrey the world would no longer be denied the miraculous healing powers of the Aborigine "healing tree," the Tea Tree—*Melaleuca alternifolia.*

A GROWTH INDUSTRY

By the start of the Second World War, Tea Tree oil from the *Melaleuca alternifolia* had earned its reputation as a miracle healer. It was medically recognized world-wide for the successful treatment of a whole range of conditions including:

- Ear, nose and throat infections: tonsillitis, gingivitis, pyorrhea, etc.
- Gynecological infections: candida, thrush, etc.
- Nail infections: paronychia, tinea, etc.
- Skin infections: impetigo, pediculosis, ringworm, etc.
- And a wide range of other contagious and non-contagious fungal, bacterial and parasitic infections (It was considered especially effective for pus filled and dirty infections.)
- Dental nerve capping
- Hemorrhages, wounds, first aid, etc.
- Not to mention all of the many and varied veterinary applications.[1]

A bottle of Tea Tree oil was a standard Government Issue in Australian Army and Navy first aid kits, especially for those soldiers serving in tropical countries. It was initially used in munitions factories to inhibit the high air-borne bacteria count. Then it was found that, by adding it to the machine cutting oils, it substantially reduced infections, especially those from abrasions caused by the off-shoot of metal filings. The production of Tea Tree oil was considered of such great importance that bush cutters were exempt from doing national service.

Surgeons, doctors, dentists, vets, and even housewives were utilizing its many healing properties. The Australian division of Colgate-Palmolive manufactured a Tea Tree oil "germicidal" soap that was very popular for a number of years.

During this meteoric rise in popularity, the actual Tea Tree industry was very modest indeed, with just over twenty steam distillation units (stills) in the Bungawalbyn area, and those were mostly small family run

1 Penfold, A.R. and Morrison, F.R. "Some Notes on the Essential Oil of *Melaleuca alternifolia,*" *Australian Journal of Pharmacy,* 18, 274-5, 1937.

businesses. The cutting and harvesting was completed totally by hand, mainly from trees growing wild in the swampy bush lands. Successful harvesting depended wholly upon manpower against the harsh elements of the Australian climate and the many hazards of working alongside the carnivorous and poisonous wildlife. Inevitably demand became far greater than supply. Throughout the war years all available stocks of good quality Tea Tree oil were taken under government control. There was little or none left for the developing marketplace. Scientists concocted cheaper synthetic alternatives. Although not as effective as Tea Tree oil, for their germicidal qualities, they were much more readily available. In the post war era the pure oil of the *Melaleuca alternifolia* was almost impossible to buy.

Right up until the middle of the 1940's the pure Tea Tree oil was still highly regarded and sought after. It had been the heyday of the Tea Tree oil industry.

During the earlier years, as the popularity of Tea Tree oil was growing, so too was medical technology. In 1928, Scottish biologist Alexander Fleming first observed the effect of penicillin on bacteria, and the antibiotic was "born." By 1941, the drug was developed and on its way to becoming established. By the 1950s it was heralded as the new "wonder drug." It was the age of synthetic and semi-synthetic medicine. Infections that were usually fatal were now virtually wiped out—tuberculosis, pneumonia, and venereal disease to name but a few. There was now hope where there had been despair. The new drugs went from strength to strength. Everyone wanted them, and everyone got them. Antibiotics were the theme of the day, and man rejoiced in the fact that he had finally triumphed over nature. The Tea Tree industry went into steep decline as natural remedies were classed as quack cures. Modern medicine was being built on synthetic chemicals and, for more than a decade, they reigned supreme.

Unfortunately the developing drug manufacturers were not interested in natural or preventive medicine, or indeed actually curing non-pathogenic diseases. The "BIG" money was in controlling symptoms so that the sufferers would be using a drug for the rest of their lives. Yes, there were side effects, but there were more drugs to control the side effects. Big money spawned big power. The press was courted, and the diminishing herbal medicine sector was held firmly down. Fortunately, as the saying goes, "You can fool some of the people some of the time, but you can never fool all of the people all of the time."

In the 1960's the "hippie" revolution started. Suddenly there was a growing awareness and unease concerning the whole scenario. Chemical pollution, animal testing, cover-ups, the addictions to synthetic drugs, and the hazardous side effects all added to the rumblings of disquiet. Then came a bombshell—an emergence of the "superbugs." Virulent strains of pathogens had evolved and were becoming immune to the antibiotics. It was clear that within the next few years these new strains could infect the population as before. With the dubious environmental and social implications all this held, once more, people were beginning to look for alternatives. "Natural" remedies were gaining in popularity, and before long the "Herbal Renaissance" had begun.

Like the tenacious hold those newly discovered Aboriginal "healing trees" had had on their natural habitat, so too the Tea Tree oil of the *Melaleuca alternifolia* was waiting in the background, forgotten but not gone. New research work was funded and the popularity of the Tea Tree was once again starting to flourish.

The first signs of the Tea Tree revival appeared when Dr. Henry Feinblatt published his work in the *Journal of the National Medical Association* (USA) in January of 1960. It was a favorable study about the action of a "Cajeput-type oil for the treatment of Furunculosis"(boils).[2] Two years later, Dr. Eduardo F. Peña (USA) completed a successful study of 130 women entitled "*Melaleuca alternifolia* Oil—Its use for Trichomonal Vaginitis and Other Vaginal Infections."[3] In April 1972, Dr. Morton Walker published the results of a study entitled "Clinical Investigation of Australian *Melaleuca alternifolia* for a Variety of Common Foot Problems" (Tinea pedis, Bromidrosis, corns, bunions, etc.) in the *Journal of Current Podiatry.*[4]

As word spread from journals to newspapers, a slowly increasing demand for both information, and indeed for the oil itself, started to grow. Articles appeared in such publications as the *Perfumer & Flavorist* [5] the *Planta Medica,*[6] the *Manufacturing Chemist,*[7] etc. The perfume and cosmetic industries and the botanical and medical faculties were just beginning to take a renewed, albeit cautious, interest.

The ups and downs of what was little more than a bush industry meant that during the 1970's the Tea Trees were still being harvested by hand from the snake and spider infested wet-lands around the Bungawalbyn Creek.

---

2 Feinblatt, H.M. "Cajeput Type Oil (Tea Tree oil) for the Treatment of Furunculosis" (boils), *Journal of the National Medical Association* USA, 52: 32-4, 1960.

3 Peña, E.F. "*Melaleuca alternifolia*: Its Use for *Trichomonal vaginitis* and Other Vaginal Infections," *Obstetrics and Gynecology,* 19:6, 793-795, 1962.

4 Walker, M. "Clinical Investigation of Australian *Melaleuca alternifolia* oil for a Variety of Common Foot Problems," *Current Podiatry,* April 7th to 15th, 1972.

5 Beylier, M.F. "Bacteriostatic Activity of Some Australian Essential Oils," *Perfumer and Flavorist International,* V4, 23-5, 1979.

6 Low, D., Rowal, B.D. and Griffin W.J. "Antibacterial Action of the Essential Oils of Some of Australian Myrtaceae," *Planta Medica,* 26, 184-189, 1974.

7 Pickering, G.B. "Cedarwood Oil Compounds, Silica Gel Separation and Tea Tree Oil as Nutmeg Substitute," *Manufacturing Chemist,* 27, 105-6, 1956.

The cutters used machete-like knives to hack off the leaves and the terminal branches, which were then transported out of the swamp to the stills. Many of the wide-tired trucks could not even attempt to make a track through the dense undergrowth, so the cutters themselves manually carried their yield out of the swamps to the awaiting transport. On a good day, one skilled worker could cut and load a truck with up to one ton of leaves and twigs.

Arriving at their destination the cuttings would then be emptied into a container over one of the large distilling vats. Using a simple wood fired steam-distillation method, these vats were fired up and allowed to reach boiling point. The resulting steam would pass through the leaves and twigs, bursting the oil bearing sacs and vaporizing the oil. The vapors then were condensed, mixed with the distillation water in the collection tank, and the pure oil was siphoned off into drums. Each standard vat could quite easily be filled by one skilled cutter and yield around 7-10 liters of pure oil. Depending on the quality of the cuttings, the process could be repeated several times until the last drop of oil had been fully extracted.

As demand was once again on the increase, so too, the Tea Tree industry itself started to rapidly expand, and inevitably the natural stands of Tea Trees were being systematically destroyed along with the associated eco-systems. It was obvious that something had to be done. So by the start of the 1980's farms were set up. Tea Trees were now being cultivated on the fertile farmlands and the oil was produced on a semi-commercial scale. From the late 1980's sustainable plantations were established and mechanical cutting was introduced. Tea Tree oil production was substantially increased to meet the ever-growing demand for high quality oil.

During this time new research work was being funded, and in 1985, Dr. Paul Belaiche completed three studies at the University of Paris, France on the use of *Melaleuca alternifolia* for the treatments of (1) Candida albicans, (2) Cystitis (urinary tract infections), and (3) Paronychia (Pus infections of the skin and nail bed). All three trials proved a success for the continued use of Tea Tree oil, and his results were supported by a number of doctors.[8, 9, 10]

More and more positive studies started to appear, like one on oral pathogens in periodontal disease by Walsh and Longstaff, published in

---

8 Belaiche, P. "Treatment of Vaginal Infections of Candida albicans with the Essential Oil of *Melaleuca alternifolia*- Cheel," *Phytotherapy*, 15, 13-14, 1985.

9 Belaiche, P. "Treatment of Chronic Urinary Tract Infections with the Essential Oil of *Melaleuca alternifolia* - Cheel," *Phytotherapy*, 15, 9-12, 1985.

10 Belaiche, P. "Treatment of Skin and Nail Infections with the Essential Oil of *Melaleuca alternifolia* - Cheel," *Phytotherapy*, 15, 15-18, 1985.

Periodontology in 1987.[11] And another in 1988 by Williams and Home, "The Composition and Bacteriocidal Activity of the Oil of *Melaleuca alternifolia*."[12] And two others by P.M. Altman; "Australian Tea Tree oil," in 1988[13] and "Australian Tea Tree Oil—a Natural Antiseptic," in 1989.[14] Over the next few years there began a whole plethora of Tea Tree studies, some pilot, some in-vitro, and others clinical. Applications were being tested and tried all over the globe.

In October 1990, Bassett, Pannowitz, and Barnetson published a clinical, double-blind comparison of the efficacy of 5% Tea Tree oil to 5% benzoyl peroxide in the *Medical Journal of Australia*. The results prompted the comments, "Both had a significant effect in ameliorating (improving) the patients' acne ... encouragingly fewer side effects were experienced by the patients treated with Tea Tree oil."[15]

In 1994, a study by Buck, Nidorf, and Addino, "Comparison of Two Topical Preparations for the Treatment of Onychomycosis: *Melaleuca alternifolia* (Tea Tree oil) and Clotrimazole" was completed. It concluded that Tea Tree oil was as effective, if not more so, as the Clotrimazole treatment for nail bed fungus.[16] Medical practitioners were beginning to notice the "good effects" on a variety of ailments including abrasions, abscesses, acne, athletes foot, canker sores, chicken pox, dandruff, eczema, hemorrhoids, head lice, infections (ear, nose, and throat), psoriasis, stings and bites, shingles, wounds, etc.

Since the beginning of the 1990's a scientific research team, led by associate Professor Tom V. Riley (including C.F. Carson and K.A. Hammer) at the Microbiology Department of the University of Western Australia, has published many papers and letters, and is continuing to study the anti-microbial properties of *Melaleuca alternifolia*. Their most notable laboratory based studies and subsequent papers include the following:

In 1993, a review into the history and unique anti-microbial properties of this ancient aboriginal oil.[17]

In 1994, two studies were published. The first was a study into the

---

11 Walsh, L.J. and Longstaff, J. "The Antimicrobial Effects of an Essential Oil on Selected Oral Pathogens," *Periodontology*, V8, 11-15, 1987.

12 Williams, L.R., Home, V.N., Zhang, X. and Stevenson, I. "The Composition and Bacteriocidal Activity of Oil of *Melaleuca alternifolia*," *International Journal of Aromatherapy*, 1:3, 15-17, 1988.

13 Altman, P.M. "Australian Tea Tree Oil," *Australian Journal of Pharmacy*, 69, 276-78, 1988.

14 Altman, P.M. "Australian Tea Tree Oil - A Natural Antiseptic," *Australian Journal of Biotechnology*, 3:4, 247-8, 1989.

15 Bassett, I.B., Pannowitz, D.L. and Barnetson, R.St.C. "A Comparative Study of Tea Tree Oil Versus Benzoyl Peroxide in the Treatment of Acne," *Medical Journal of Australia*, 153:8, 455-458, 1990.

16 Buck, D.S., Nidorf, D.M. and Addino, J.G. "Comparison of Two Topical Preparations for the Treatment of Onychomycosis: *Melaleuca alternifolia* (Tea Tree Oil) and Clotrimazole," *Journal of Family Practice*, 38, 601-5, 1994.

17 Carson, C.F. and Riley, T.V. "Antimicrobial Activity of the Essential Oil of *Melaleuca alternifolia* (A Review)," *Letters in Applied Microbiology*, 16, 49-55, 1993.

unique anti-bacterial properties of Tea Tree oil.[18] The second was a positive study into the effect of Tea Tree oil on the bacteria that can cause acne and related problems.[19]

During 1995 four studies were published. The first, and most important to mankind, was an in-vitro study into how Tea Tree oil can inhibit and destroy the bacteria that has become immune to methicillin, an antibiotic normally used to combat the *Staphylococcus aureus* species of gram-positive bacteria. Hospitals all over the world are finding more and more isolates of *Staphylococci* that are becoming immune to the once effective drugs. This study successfully showed that all sixty-six isolates were susceptible to the oil of *Melaleuca alternifolia* even at a quite low dilution.[20]

The next study that year detailed a broth micro-dilution method that could effectively be used to detect the susceptibilities of *E. Coli* and *Staphylococcus aureus.*[21]

The third in 1995 was a study into eight of the major components that make up the unique composition of Tea Tree oil, including Terpinen 4-ol and Cineole, etc. This is extremely useful for all sectors of the Tea Tree industry, helping to determine the best possible composition of an oil for medicinal effectiveness, etc.[22]

The final study that year took a critical look at the toxicity of Tea Tree oil, opening the way to discovering which components cause a reaction in those who are susceptible.[23]

In 1996, an in-vitro study showed that Tea Tree oil could inhibit the pathogenic bacteria that inhabits the skin's surface but could, in turn, still maintain the essential skin flora. This had good implications for using a low dilution in personal care products and skin creams.[24]

Also in 1996 an important study into the effectiveness of Tea Tree oil against the various gram-positive *Streptococcus spp. Streptococci* bacteria is implicated in many lesser (group B) and major, sometimes fatal, (group A)

---

18 Carson, C.F. and Riley, T.V. "The Antimicrobial Activity of Tea Tree Oil," *Medical Journal of Australia,*160, 236, 1994.

19 Carson, C.F. and Riley, T.V. "Susceptibility of *Propionibacterium acnes* to the Essential Oil of *Melaleuca alternifolia,*" *Letters in Applied Microbiology,* 19, 24-25, 1994.

20 Carson, C.F., Cookson, B.D., Farrelly, H.D. and Riley, T.V. "Susceptibility of Methicillin-resistant *Staphylococcus aureus* to the Essential Oil *Melaleuca alternifolia,*" *Journal of Antimicrobial Chemotherapy,* 35:3, 421-4, 1995.

21 Carson, C.F., Hammer, K.A. and Riley T.V. "Broth Micro-dilution Method for Determining the Susceptibility of *Escherichia coli* (*E coli*) and *Staphylococcus aureus* to the Essential Oil of *Melaleuca alternifolia,*" *Microbios,* 82, 181-185, 1995.

22 Carson, C.F. and Riley, T.V. "Antimicrobial Activity of the Major Components of the Essential Oil of *Melaleuca alternifolia,*" *Journal of Applied Bacteriology,* 78:3, 264-9, 1995.

23 Carson, C.F. and Riley, T.V. "Toxicity of the Essential Oil of *Melaleuca alternifolia* (or Tea Tree Oil)," (Letter) *Journal of Toxicology-Clinical Toxicology,* 33:2, 193-4, 1995.

24 Hammer, K.A., Carson, C.F. and Riley, T.V. "Susceptibility of Transient and Commensal Skin Flora to the Essential Oil of *Melaleuca alternifolia* (Tea Tree Oil)," *American Journal of Infection Control,* 24:3, 186-9, 1996.

infections including Strep Throat and the flesh eating *Necrotizing fasciitis* (Type II).[25]

In 1997, their in-vitro study found that Tea Tree oil could inhibit the fungi *Malassezia furfur* (formally known as *Pityrosporum ovale*) which can contribute to dandruff and other various skin conditions.[26]

Their work in 1998 found that commercial Tea Tree products were as effective an anti-fungal agent as a Tea Tree dilution for inhibiting superficial *Candida albicans* type infections.[27]

And in the last year of this century, one of their in-vitro studies suggested that Tea Tree oil may also have a place in combating bacterial vaginosis.[28]

Two projects due to be completed soon are research into the anti-inflammatory properties and the anti-viral activity of Tea Tree oil. Various trials, projects, and medical collaborations are also in the pipeline. At last, mainly due to their invaluable in-vitro studies, things are really starting to move and are actually gathering momentum. Hopefully this will give Tea Tree oil the much needed credibility with those who choose not to see the healing of generations of people as proof of efficacy.

TEA TREE OIL APPLICATIONS– AN AMAZING ANTISEPTIC AND MUCH MUCH MORE!

In the early days of Tea Tree oil, back in the 1930's and 1940's, when the scientific evidence was in its infancy, it became clear that Tea Tree oil was a very valuable commodity. Humphrey's paper, "A New Australian Germicide," published in the *Medical Journal of Australia,* was really the catalyst that started the commercial ball rolling. Ever since the very first evidence, new testing methods, superior emulsifiers and more advanced surfactants have all helped us to understand and use Tea Tree oil in a vast array of products.[1, 2]

---

25 Carson, C.F., Hammer, K.A. and Riley, T.V. "In-vitro Activity of the Essential Oil of *Melaleuca alternifolia* Against *Streptococcus Spp.*," *Journal of Antimicrobial Chemotherapy,* 37:6, 1177-8, 1996.

26 Hammer, K.A., Carson, C.F. and Riley, T.V. "In-vitro Susceptibility of *Malassezia furfur* to the Essential Oil of *Melaleuca alternifolia,*" *Journal of Medical and Veterinary Mycology,* 35:5, 375-7, 1997.

27 Hammer, K.A., Carson, C.F. and Riley, T.V. "In-vitro Activity of Essential Oils, in Particular *Melaleuca alternifolia* (Tea Tree Oil and Tea Tree Oil Products) Against *Candida spp.*," *Journal of Antimicrobial Chemotherapy,* 42:5, 591-5, 1998.

28 Hammer, K.A., Carson, C.F. and Riley, T.V. "In-vitro Susceptibilities of *Lactobacilli* and Organisms Associated with Bacterial Vaginosis to *Melaleuca alternifolia* (Tea Tree oil)," (Letter) *Antimicrobial Agents and Chemotherapy,* Jan 1999.

---

1 Williams, L.R., Home, V.N. and Asre, S. "Antimicrobial Activity of Oil of *Melaleuca alternifolia.* Its Potential Use in Cosmetics and Toiletries," *Cosmetics, Aerosols & Toiletries in Australia,* 4:4, 1990.

2 Altman, P.M. "Australian Tea Tree Oil," *Australian Journal of Pharmacy,* 69, 276-78, 1988.

ANTIBACTERIAL SOAPS

The first commercially blended Tea Tree oil product was an antiseptic soap, which was manufactured by the Australian division of Colgate-Palmolive. The soap all but disappeared after the war years with the rise in synthetic disinfectants. In the early 1980's antiseptic soaps, creams and lotions started to emerge on a wider scale. A positive trial conducted by The Associated Foodstuff Laboratories of Australia in 1983 showed that the bacterial count on hands was substantially reduced by washing with Tea Tree products. Dr. Humphrey had long advocated the use of its superior germicidal action, and many other clinical trials have later confirmed this.[3, 4, 5]

ACNE CREAMS AND LOTIONS

Many people suffer from acne and facial boils at some time in their lives. There have been quite a few positive trials using Tea Tree oil in various products for these conditions. The unique penetrating action of the Tea Tree oil helps to rid the dermal layers of the invading bacteria. A soon to be friend of mine who had four boils on her chin and was at her wits end contacted us to ask our advice. She had been on antibiotics for over three months, but the boils were still thriving. We suggested she use a Tea Tree problem skin lotion, so she went back to her doctor who agreed to take her off the antibiotics. Within two weeks, two of the boils had disappeared and the third was shrinking fast. Within one month she had just a faint mark where the last boil had finally admitted defeat. She was amazed with the results. We had seen it all before![6,7,8]

MOISTURIZING CREAMS & LOTIONS

Although very few clinical studies have been completed in this area, there is much anecdotal evidence detailing the good effects of Tea Tree oil, applied in creams and lotions, to help alleviate skin conditions such as psoriasis and eczema, etc. A large Australian Tea Tree company has done its own investigations into inflammatory skin conditions with some quite positive results. A couple of the studies, "A Clinical Investigation of a Tea

3 Hammer, K.A., Carson, C.F. and Riley, T.V. "Susceptibility of Transient and Commensal Skin Flora to the Essential Oil of *Melaleuca alternifolia* (Tea Tree Oil)," *American Journal of Infection Control,* 24:3, 186-9, 1996.

4 Beylier, M.F. "Bacteriostatic Activity of Some Australian Essential Oils," *Perfumer and Flavorist International,* V4:23-5, 1979.

5 Williams, L.R., Home, V.N. and Asre, S. "Antimicrobial Activity of Oil of *Melaleuca alternifolia.* Its Potential Use in Cosmetics and Toiletries," *Cosmetics, Aerosols & Toiletries in Australia,* 4:4, 1990.

6 Bassett, I.B., Pannowitz, D.L. and Barnetson, R.St.C. "A Comparative Study of Tea Tree Oil Versus Benzoyl Peroxide in the Treatment of Acne," *Medical Journal of Australia,* 153:8, 455-458, 1990.

7 Carson, C.F. and Riley, T.V. "Susceptibility of *Propionibacterium acnes* to the Essential Oil of *Melaleuca alternifolia,*" *Letters in Applied Microbiology,* 19, 24-25, 1994.

8 Feinblatt, H.M. "Cajeput Type Oil (Tea Tree oil) for the Treatment of Furunculosis" (boils), *Journal of the National Medical Association* (USA), 52, 32-4, 1960.

Tree Oil Preparation for the Re-hydration of the Skin in Lower Limb" by Jill Fogharty, and "A Pilot Study into Australian Tea Tree Oil" by M. Abdulla, have been successfully completed. Where local inflammation is present due to skin complaints, stings, bites, etc., Tea Tree oil in dilution was effective in soothing local irritation and pain. The best thing about Tea Tree moisturizing creams and lotions is that, even with a quite low dilution of Tea Tree oil, they can inhibit harmful bacteria while maintaining the resident skin flora.[9,10]

ORAL/DENTAL PRODUCTS

An article in one of Australia's popular health magazines (*Prevention* January 1992), and written by Dr. William Mayo, stated that Tea Tree oil was effectively used in many oral preparations (toothpastes, mouthwashes, lip salves, sore throat sprays, lozenges, cold sore ointments, etc). There have been many clinical studies on oral pathogens. Tea tree oil is second to none for helping to keep teeth healthy and white, or to guard against mouth infections.

Dr. Andrew Weil, the well-known medical author and physician, frequently recommends Tea Tree oil toothpastes and mouthwashes for a number of oral problems. Some of these include halitosis (bad breath), gum disease, and canker sores.[11, 12, 13, 14]

HAIR CARE PRODUCTS

Tea Tree oil is a very effective ingredient in shampoos and conditioners. It helps to keep the hair and scalp in tiptop condition. It was reported as early as 1939 that Tea Tree oil was an excellent ingredient in soaps and shampoos. An Australian chemist advertised the use of a 3% Tea Tree shampoo for the treatment of dandruff. Today *Melaleuca alternifolia* has finally been clinically sanctioned as a possible anti-dandruff shampoo ingredient, and shown that, even at a quite low dilution, it can inhibit the yeast that causes the problem.[15,16]

---

9 Hammer, K.A., Carson, C.F. and Riley, T.V. "Susceptibility of Transient and Commensal Skin Flora to the Essential Oil of *Melaleuca alternifolia* (Tea Tree Oil)," *American Journal of Infection Control,* 24:3, 186-9, 1996.

10 Shemesh, A. and Mayo, W.L. "A Natural Antiseptic and Fungicide," *International Journal of Alternative and Complementary Medicine,* Dec. 1991.

11 Shemesh, A. and Mayo, W.L. "A Natural Antiseptic and Fungicide," *International Journal of Alternative and Complementary Medicine,* Dec. 1991.

12 Walsh, L.J. and Longstaff, J. "The Antimicrobial Effects of an Essential Oil on Selected Oral Pathogens," *Periodontology,* V8, 11-15, 1987.

13 Shapiro, S., Meier, A. and Guggenheim, B. "The Anti-microbial Activity of Essential Oils and Essential Oil Components Towards Oral Bacteria," *Oral Microbiolog. Immunology* (Denmark), 9:4, 202-8, 1994.

14 Weil, A. *Ask Dr. Weil,* http://cgi.pathfinder.com/drweil

15 Goldsborough, R.E. "Ti-Tree Oil," *The Manufacturing Chemist,* 57-58-60, Feb 1939.

16 Hammer, K.A., Carson, C.F. and Riley, T.V. "In-vitro Susceptibility of *Malassezia furfur* to the Essential Oil of *Melaleuca alternifolia,*" *Journal of Medical and Veterinary Mycology,* 35:5, 375-7, 1997.

PARASITICIDE AND INSECT REPELLENT

There are many anecdotal cases of Tea Tree oil soothing pain and itching after a sting or an insect bite. The analgesic qualities together with its powerful solvent action (dissipating the venom) is probably what makes it so effective. It is also thought that the solvent properties help to dissolve the hard outer case of the insect and so making it an effective insecticide/parasiticide, while the Terpenes present in the oil act as an insect repellent.

Tea Tree has been used for a number of years by doctors for the safe removal of parasites. With the growing concern over the safety of prescription lotions, it was refreshing to actually hear a qualified doctor give his approval. The well-known physician and medical author, Dr. Andrew Weil, recommends the use of Tea Tree oil and other oils for the treatment of head lice. [17,18,19,20]

ANTIFUNGAL CREAMS AND FOOT CARE PRODUCTS

Tea Tree oil is very effective on all sorts of foot problems and infections. Many successful trials have been carried out in this area, from athletes foot (Tinea pedis) and ringworm, to warts, even on rough and cracked skin. It is used by podiatrists all over the world.

On his Web site, *Ask Dr. Weil*, the highly respected medical author writes, "Tea Tree oil is the best treatment I know for fungal infections of the skin (athlete's foot, ringworm, jock itch). It will also clear up fungal infections of the toenails or fingernails, a condition notoriously resistant to treatment, even by strong systemic antibiotics."[21]

We have a lovely letter from a parent whose son's feet were so badly infected with Plantar warts that his doctor had said that surgery was the only option. We put her in touch with a podiatrist who we knew used Tea Tree oil on his patients. After a few weeks of treatment, the son was well on his way to a complete recovery, and without the intervention of surgery.[22,23,24]

---

17 Veal, L. "The Potential Effectiveness of Essential Oils as a Treatment for Head Lice, *Pediculus Humanus Capitis*," *Complementary Ther. Nurs. Midwifery*, 2:4, 97-101, 1996.

18 McDonald, L.G. and Tovey, E. "The Effectiveness of Benzyl Benzoate and Some Essential Oils as Laundry Additives for Killing House Dustmites," *Journal Allergy and Clinical Immunology*, 1993.

19 Williams, L.R., Home, V.N. and Asre S. "Antimicrobial Activity of Oil of *Melaleuca alternifolia*. Its Potential Use in Cosmetics and Toiletries," *Cosmetics, Aerosols & Toiletries in Australia*, 4:4, 1990.

20 Weil, A. *Ask Dr. Weil*, http://cgi.pathfinder.com/drweil

21 Weil, A. *Ask Dr. Weil*, http://cgi.pathfinder.com/drweil

22 Tong M.M., Altman, P.M. and Barnetson R.St.C. "Tea Tree Oil in the Treatment of Tinea pedis," *Australian Journal of Dermatology*, 33:3, 145-9, 1992.

23 Walker, M. "Clinical Investigation of Australian *Melaleuca alternifolia* oil for a Variety of Common Foot Problems," *Current Podiatry*, April 7th to 15th, 1972.

24 Nenoff, P., et al. "Antifungal Activity of the Essential Oil of *Melaleuca alternifolia* (Tea Tree oil) Against Pathogenic Fungi In-vitro," *Skin Pharmacology*, 9:6, 388-394, 1996.

PERSONAL CARE PRODUCTS

Tea Tree oil products for personal care are gathering momentum. Dr. Humphrey in his writings of 1930 stated that it was a good deodorant, killing the bacteria that produced the odor. Hammer et al found that, at low dilution, it could be used on the skin and still maintain resident skin flora. Today we have a far wider choice of personal care items, as word of the effectiveness of this wonderful oil spreads far and wide. From deodorant to body lotion, cosmetics, sunscreen, hand cream, to aftershave lotion, after-sun cream and bubble bath, its non-sting healing properties are being utilized as never before.[25,26]

VAGINAL DOUCHES AND GENITAL CREAMS

Unfortunately for us humans, we have many sites that can harbor the pathogenic yeasts and bacteria that cause infection. Central heating, synthetic underwear, tight-fitting clothes, etc., all add to the problem. Fortunately there are many Tea Tree personal hygiene products on the market with plenty of clinical trials to back up the claims that Tea Tree oil can effectively reduce harmful parasites that thrive in dark, warm places on the body. Dr. Andrew Weil claims that, for vaginal yeast infections, Tea Tree oil "is at least as effective as the usual prescription remedy."[27,28,29,30]

INFLAMMATION

Again this is another area where Tea Tree oil has been used for decades by alternative practitioners in the treatment of inflammation and pain. From insect bite salves to rheumatic rubs and sports care products, there is much anecdotal evidence to support its use in this area. The first clinical evidence that Tea Tree oil may be able to reduce inflammation and associated pain has been found in a study by the College of Dentistry at the University of Tennessee Memphis.[31] The Rural Industries Research and Development Corporation (RIRDC) in Australia has funded further research into this and the results should be published soon.

---

25 Altman, P.M. "Australian Tea Tree Oil - An Update," *Cosmetics, Aerosols & Toiletries in Australia,* 5:4, 27-9, 1991.

26 Priest, D. "Tea Tree Oil in Cosmetics- The Promise and the Proof," (Technical paper) *Cosmetics, Aerosols & Toiletries in Australia,* 9:4, 1995.

27 Weil, A. *Ask Dr. Weil,* http://cgi.pathfinder.com/drweil

28 Peña, E.F. "*Melaleuca alternifolia:* Its Use for Trichomonal vaginitis and Other Vaginal Infections," *Obstetrics and Gynecology,* 19:6, 793-795, 1962.

29 Hammer, K.A., Carson, C.F. and Riley, T.V. "In-vitro Activity of Essential Oils, in Particular *Melaleuca alternifolia* (Tea Tree Oil and Tea Tree Oil Products) against *Candida spp.,*" *Journal of Antimicrobial Chemotherapy,* 42:5, 591-5, 1998.

30 Hammer, K.A., Carson, C.F. and Riley, T.V. "In-vitro Susceptibilities of *Lactobacilli* and Organisms Associated with Bacterial Vaginosis to *Melaleuca alternifolia* (Tea Tree oil)," (Letter) *Antimicrobial Agents and Chemotherapy,* Jan 1999.

31 Dabbous, K.H., Pippin, M.A., Pabst, K.M., Pabst, M.J. and Haney, L. "Superoxide Release by Neutrophils is Inhibited by Tea Tree Oil," (Supported by NIDR DEO5494) College of Dentistry, UT Memphis, 1993.

BURN GELS

There is a great deal of anecdotal (but not very much scientific) evidence that Tea Tree gel helps to alleviate pain and infection when applied to burns. Many leading Tea Tree companies are using the oil of *Melaleuca alternifolia* in a whole range of new and innovative burn gels and impregnated dressings. The water soluble gel helps to quickly cool down the burn while the Melaleuca oil, held in suspension, reduces the pain and inflammation. Healing is accelerated with much less likelihood of infection and scarring—great news for casualty units, fire departments, industry, schools, families, and in fact, anyone who is likely to treat burns and scalds.

Did you know? It was reported that Australian actor Mel Gibson insisted on using Tea Tree impregnated fire blankets on the set during the filming of the amazing fire scenes for the film Braveheart, just in case any of the actors or film crew were accidentally burned! Nice one Mel!

HAND & NAIL CARE

Dr. E.M. Humphrey in the 1930's found that "The pus solvent properties of Tea Tree oil made it an excellent application for the fungal nail disease paronychia, which if left untreated could result in the deformity and eventual loss of the nail." Dr. Andrew Weil claims that Tea Tree oil works better, and is much cheaper, than prescription antifungals for fungal infections of the toenails or fingernails.[32,33,34,35]

COUGHS, COLDS & FLU

Alternative practitioners have successfully used Tea Tree oil in sprays (for strep throat), inhalations and decongestant chest rubs. There is some evidence available in peer-reviewed journals that can collaborate these facts, but more research needs to be done in this area.[36,37,38]

THE FIRST ANTI-VIRAL EVIDENCE

Most alternative practitioners have known that Tea Tree oil of *Melaleuca alternifolia* has shown signs of anti-viral activity, especially with the Herpes virus (cold sores, chicken pox and shingles blisters,

32 Penfold, A.R. and Morrison, F.R. "Some Notes on the Essential Oil of *Melaleuca alternifolia*," *Australian Journal of Pharmacy*, 18, 274-5, 1937.

33 Humphrey, E.M. "A New Australian Germicide," *Medical Journal of Australia*, I, 417-418, 1930.

34 Buck, D.S, Nidorf, D.M. and Addino, J.G. "Comparison of Two Topical Preparations for the Treatment of Onychomycosis: *Melaleuca alternifolia* (Tea Tree Oil) and Clotrimazole," *Journal of Family Practice*, 38, 601-5, 1994.

35 Weil, A. *Ask Dr. Weil*, http://cgi.pathfinder.com/drweil

36 Carson, C.F., Hammer, K.A. and Riley, T.V. "In-vitro Activity of the Essential Oil of *Melaleuca alternifolia* against *Streptococcus Spp.*," *Journal of Antimicrobial Chemotherapy*, 37:6, 1177-8, 1996.

37 Coutts, M. "The Bronchoscopic Treatment of Bronchiectasis," *Medical Journal Australia*, July 1937.

38 Shemesh, A. and Mayo, W.L. "A Natural Antiseptic and Fungicide," *International Journal of Alternative and Complementary Medicine*, Dec. 1991.

warts, etc.). Now that the first research report completed by Chris Bishop at John Moores University, Liverpool, UK, has been published, others supported by the Rural Industries Research and Development Corporation (RIRDC) are set to follow.[39]

AT WAR WITH THE SUPERBUGS

Methicillin-resistant *Staphylococcus aureus* (MRSA, Golden-staph, Super-staph) is believed to be at epidemic proportions. The last of the synthesized antibiotics are becoming increasingly less effective against it. Tea Tree oil, at a low dilution of less than 2%, is proving to be the one last hope. Unfortunately, because Tea Tree oil cannot be patented or held exclusive, large pharmaceutical companies do not see the need to help with research. Could this mean that they are more interested in profits than in people's health? [40,41,42,43]

CHILD CARE

There are many safe, dermatologically tested Tea Tree products available that are designed for children. It is comforting to know that Tea Tree is still a very effective pathogenic bacteria inhibitor even at a low dilution of 0.25% in some cases.[44]

PET CARE

The beneficial effects of Tea Tree oil apply to animals as well. Skin problems, wounds, insect bites and stings, and ringworm can all be treated very successfully with the oil or products made with the oil. One property of Tea Tree oil in particular is very beneficial to pets—it is a very effective insect repellent. It's a useful treatment and deterrent for fleas, ticks, and mites.[45,46]

---

39 Bishop, C.D. "Anti-viral Activity of the Essential Oil of *Melaleuca alternifolia* (Maiden & Betche) Cheel (Tea Tree) Against Tobacco Mosaic Virus," (Research Report) *Journal of Essential Oil Research*, 7, 641-644, 1995.

40 Carson, C.F., Cookson, B.D., Farrelly, H.D. and Riley, T.V. "Susceptibility of Methicillin-resistant *Staphylococcus aureus* to the Essential Oil *Melaleuca alternifolia*," *Journal of Antimicrobial Chemotherapy*, 35:3, 421-4, 1995.

41 Carson, C.F., Hammer, K.A. and Riley, T.V. "Broth Micro-dilution Method for Determining the Susceptibility of *Escherichia coli* (E coli) and *Staphylococcus aureus* to the Essential Oil of *Melaleuca alternifolia*," *Microbios*, 82:332, 181-185, 1995.

42 Carson, C.F., Riley, T.V. and Cookson, B.D. "Efficacy and Safety of Tea Tree Oil as a Topical Antimicrobial Agent," (editorial) *Journal of Hospital Infection*, 40:3, 175-8, 1998.

43 Elsom, G. "Susceptibility of Methicillin-resistant *Staphylococcus aureus* to Tea Tree Oil and Mupirocin," *Journal of Antimicrobial Chemotherapy*, V43, 427-428, 1999.

44 Hammer, K.A., Carson, C.F. and Riley, T.V. "Susceptibility of Transient and Commensal Skin Flora to the Essential Oil of *Melaleuca alternifolia* (Tea Tree Oil)," *American Journal of Infection Control*, 24:3, 186-9, 1996.

45 Carson, C.F. and Riley, T.V. "Toxicity of the Essential Oil of *Melaleuca alternifolia* (or Tea Tree Oil)," (Letter) *Journal of Toxicology-Clinical Toxicology*, 33:2, 193-4, 1995.

46 Southwell, I., Markham, J. and Mann, C. "Why Cineole is Not Detrimental to Tea Tree Oil," *Rural Industries Research and Development Corporation*, Research Paper Series 97/54, 1997.

AGRICULTURAL APPLICATIONS

Although there have not been a great deal of clinical studies on the use of Tea Tree oil in agriculture, its anti-fungal, parasiticidal, and indeed, anti-viral properties can be utilized for use in the greenhouse and garden (see the first anti-viral evidence above). Australian farmers and organic growers have been using Tea Tree products for a number of years.[47,48]

HOUSEHOLD CLEANING & LAUNDRY

The solvent properties of Tea Tree oil, which are so useful at dissolving pus and debris in wounds, are also brilliant in household cleaning products and in the laundry. Today, companies all around the globe are utilizing its unique solvent and anti-microbial qualities. There are soaps, stain removers, fabric softeners, laundry detergents and whiteners, copper and brass cleaners, dish detergents, window cleaners, all-purpose cleaners, bathroom cleaners, furniture polish, air fresheners, odor eliminators, floor cleaners, hospital grade disinfectants, etc. Tea Tree oil can also be used very effectively as an anti-microbial surface cleaner. It is many times more "active" than a comparable strength disinfectant.[49,50]

The household of the 21st Century has a unique opportunity to say "No!" to those harsh synthetic chemicals that are slowly poisoning our planet. While we still have natural, biodegradable commodities like the oil of the Melaleuca alternifolia we have a choice—a greener choice that can not only assist in healing our bodies, but can also safely cleanse all around our homes too, quite literally from basement to attic.

A LESSON IN QUALITY

With the spreading world-wide popularity of Tea Tree oil, there was inevitably a growing demand for high quality oil with consistent healing properties. Unfortunately, less scrupulous companies could easily sell an inferior oil, trading solely on the good reputation earned by the pure oil of *Melaleuca alternifolia*. With no quality standards in place, these companies could quite legally mix the pure oil with a cheaper oil, having little or no healing qualities, and market the blend as "Tea Tree oil" or "Melaleuca oil."

Even if the oil is wholly derived from the *Melaleuca alternifolia* tree, this does not guarantee its therapeutic value. Tree genetics, growing conditions, distillation methods, and storage can all affect oil quality to a

---

47 Small, B.E.J. "Tea Tree Oil," *Australian Journal of Experimental Agriculture and Animal Husbandry*, V21, 1981.
48 Olsen, M.W. "Control of *Sphaerotheca fuliginea* on Cucurbits with a 1.5% Dilution of an Oil Extracted from the Australian Tea Tree," *Phytopathology*, 78:12, 1595, 1988.
49 Altman, P.M. "Australian Tea Tree Oil," *Australian Journal of Pharmacy*, 69, 276-78, 1988.
50 Altman, P.M. "Australian Tea Tree Oil - A Natural Antiseptic," *Australian Journal of Biotechnology*, 3:4 247-8, 1989.

degree. This is why, in 1967, in order to protect both the consumer and the Tea Tree industry, the Australian Standards Association established a standard for the oil.

This new standard was based on two of the oil's key components—Terpinen 4-ol and Cineole. As far back as 1925, it was known that Terpinen 4-ol was the main anti-microbial component. Obviously, higher levels of Terpinen 4-ol are desirable. Cineole is the component that gives Tea Tree oil its unique penetrating ability. But high levels of Cineole can be irritating to sensitive skin, so lower levels of Cineole are preferable. Consequently, the Australian Standards Association set the 1967 standard so that Melaleuca oil should have a minimum content of 35% Terpinen 4-ol and a maximum of 10% Cineole.

Unfortunately these new requirements led to an over-production of unmarketable oil that failed to reach the required standard. To save the ailing and discontented Tea Tree industry, the standard was relaxed in 1985 to a minimum content of 30% Terpinen 4-ol and a maximum of 15% Cineole. Fortunately for us, there are a number of reputable suppliers who still sell high-quality oil which falls well within the original (higher) standard.

Please be aware that there are many oils that technically can be called "Tea Tree oil" or "Melaleuca oil." There are over 150 species of Melaleuca trees, some with nearly identical main components, but there is only one *Melaleuca alternifolia*. To be sure that you have the authentic Australian Tea Tree oil, it must state on the label that it is the oil of the "*Melaleuca alternifolia.*" It should also contain more than 35% Terpinen 4-ol and less than 10% Cineole. It is very important to know your supplier and to make sure that the oil you purchase is of a high therapeutic grade. If in any doubt, go back to your supplier and ask to see a detailed specification. A reputable supplier would be happy to oblige. There are reputable companies today that have never lowered their standards and have always sold the pure oil of *Melaleuca alternifolia* that is well within the set guidelines.

This all reminds me of a very apt slogan I once saw:

"Nothing added, nothing removed,
Nature's best cannot be improved."

Tea Tree oil of the *Melaleuca alternifolia* is a uniquely complex substance that continues to delight and surprise us the more we learn about it. It is truly one of "nature's best," and one of nature's most potent, remarkable, and useful gifts.

CHAPTER THREE

3

Grape Seed Extract

"The most potent preventive medicine you can take!"

ABOUT THE AUTHOR, DR. CLARK HANSEN

Clark Hansen, N.M.D., is a Doctor of Naturopathic Medicine with a very busy private practice in Scottsdale, Arizona. He graduated from the John Bastyr College of Naturopathic Medicine in Seattle, Washington, in 1986. Since 1988, Dr. Hansen has served as the President and Medical Director of The Arizona Institute of Natural Medicine, a medical clinic that attracts patients from all over the U.S.

Dr. Hansen is one of the founders of the Southwest College of Naturopathic Medicine and Health Sciences in Scottsdale, Arizona, where he serves as a member of the Board of Advisors and as an Associate Professor of Clinical Medicine. Dr. Hansen is a member of the American Association of Naturopathic Physicians, the Arizona Naturopathic Medical Association, the American Holistic Medical Association, and the Physicians Committee for Responsible Medicine.

THE DISCOVERY OF A LIFETIME

Proanthocyanidin (PCO) is a natural plant bioflavonoid extracted from the seeds of grapes. Also known as Pycnogenol, this potent bioflavonoid is so essential to our existence that it should be considered a vitamin, because our bodies cannot make it and we cannot survive without it. Its healing and preventive benefits are simply phenomenal. It has been used in France for more than 40 years but has only recently been discovered by Americans. PCO has been found to be the most potent antioxidant ever discovered. It is 20 times more potent than Vitamin C and 50 times more potent than Vitamin E. It is also anti-inflammatory, anti-allergic, and anti-mutagenic. PCO bioflavonoids are found in the peels, skins, and seeds of fruits and vegetables, and the barks of certain trees, including the lemon tree, the French maritime pine tree, and the leaves of the hazelnut tree. Grape Seed Extract yields a 95% concentration of PCO, the highest of any source. Pine bark is second, with an 85% concentration.

DISCOVERY OF PCO

In 1948, Jacques Masquelier, a young Ph.D. candidate from the University of Bordeaux, France, isolated PCO from peanuts. In his doctoral thesis, Masquelier demonstrated the ability of PCO to double the strength of blood vessels within a few hours after administration to laboratory animals. In 1951, Professor Masquelier patented a PCO extract from pine bark. Nineteen years later, in 1970, he patented a second PCO extract from grape seeds which he found to yield a 10% higher concentration. In 1986, Dr. Masquelier discovered that PCO from grape seeds has an intense free radical scavenging effect. These discoveries were laid down in his U.S. Patent # 4,598,360 of October 6, 1987. After years of continued research he said, "The test showed that in this respect PCO from grape seeds has an advantage over PCO from pine bark. PCO from grape seeds contains the gallic esters of PCOs. These PCO-esters have been recently described as the most active substances in the battle against free radicals."

NATURE'S MOST POTENT ANTIOXIDANT

PCO bioflavonoids have a specific affinity for the connective tissue (collagen and elastin) of the body, providing stabilization and protection from premature breakdown. When you eat them they become incorporated into the connective tissues of your skin, blood vessels, joints, and cell membranes. They protect your body from free radical damage. Free radicals are produced from oxygen metabolism within the body and from exposure to certain chemicals, environmental pollutants, sunlight, radiation burns, cigarette smoke, drugs, alcohol, viruses, bacteria, parasites, dietary fats, and more.

Free radicals destroy cell membranes, damage collagen and other connective tissues, disrupt important physiologic processes, and create mutations in the DNA of cells. They are implicated in more than 60 diseases, including heart disease, hardening of the arteries, arthritis, Alzheimer's disease, cataracts, and cancer. Free radicals are oxygen molecules with a missing or unpaired electron which spin erratically throughout the body, damaging every tissue they bounce into until they are finally quenched by an antioxidant such as vitamin C or E, beta-carotene, bioflavonoids, or certain enzymes produced by the body. As we grow older, the body's inherent production of free radical deactivating enzymes decreases. As this happens, the skin becomes leathery and wrinkled, arteries lose their elasticity, joints and cartilage stiffen, vision becomes cloudy, the spine becomes stooped, and every part of the body gradually deteriorates. PCO prevents the cross-linking of body tissues that is associated with aging. It blocks connective tissue-destroying enzymes that otherwise would have a cumulative thinning and weakening effect on the body's connective tissue over time.

THE SECRET TO YOUTHFULNESS

PCO helps protect the skin from ultraviolet radiation damage that leads to wrinkles and skin cancer. Because it stabilizes collagen and elastin, PCO can help to improve the elasticity and youthfulness of the skin. Its potent antioxidant effect in the skin has even been found to reverse the process of pigment lipofuscin, causing unsightly age spots to fade and disappear. Many individuals taking PCO have seen it reduce the appearance of surgical scars and stretch marks.

The ability of PCO to stabilize and protect collagen and elastin within joints has demonstrated remarkable effects in the relief of pain and inflammation associated with arthritis. In clinical and experimental studies, PCO has been shown to inhibit inflammatory swelling including postoperative swelling. Many arthritis sufferers say that PCO completely eliminates stiffness and restores their mobility. It also inhibits excessive production of histamine that causes allergic disorders and the inflammatory swelling related to allergies. In fact many cases of arthritis are due to allergies.

PCO has been shown to: improve blood vessel elasticity; increase red blood cell pliability; inhibit platelet stickiness and clumping; normalize blood flow; improve oxygenation of ischemic areas; decrease bruising, bleeding and edema; prevent blood clots; and reduce elevated blood pressure. People taking Grape Seed Extract have found that it can lower their cholesterol levels remarkably, and researchers have found that PCO reduces the size of cholesterol plaque in the blood vessel walls of animals.

Patients with Multiple Sclerosis (MS), a syndrome of progressive destruction of the myelin sheath that surrounds the nerves, have reported significant improvement while taking PCO. Many studies have demonstrated that patients with MS have reduced activity of the antioxidant enzyme Glutathione peroxidase. The ability of PCO to reduce the progressive symptoms of MS may be the result of the fact that it is one of the few antioxidants that can cross the blood-brain barrier.

PCO has also been shown to protect cell membranes and thereby prevent mutations caused by damage to DNA. This may help prevent the onset of cancer. One study has shown that the risk of developing cancer is 11.4 times higher in those with low levels of the antioxidants vitamin E and Selenium. Since PCO is 50 times more potent than Vitamin E as an antioxidant, it is expected to have an even greater individual cancer-preventing effect. Additionally, PCO may work with Vitamin E to enhance the body's ability to fight and prevent cancer by protecting the cancer-fighting cells known as *natural killer cells*. PCO is also known to work synergistically with Vitamin C to increase the longevity of *natural killer cells*.

Due to its protective effects on connective tissue within the eye, PCO is effective in stopping the progression of cataracts and reversing glaucoma and age-related macular degeneration, the leading cause of blindness.

Grape Seed Extract is the most potent preventive nutrient you can buy. It can prevent the cross-linking of your connective tissue, promote new collagen and elastin production, and slow down or reverse the biological process of aging to help prevent heart disease, cancer, strokes, diabetes, cataracts, glaucoma, arthritis, allergies, wrinkles, cellulite, and more.

Bioavailability: PCO is water soluble, readily absorbed within 60 minutes, and actively circulates in the body for three days. Unlike most antioxidants, PCO can even cross the blood-brain barrier.

Safety: PCO is nontoxic, noncarcinogenic, non-teratogenic. It has been thoroughly tested in France for more than 40 years and used by more than 10 million people. Because grape seeds are so bitter, occasional nausea or stomach upset has been reported.

Dosage: Take 50 mg to 300 mg per day depending on intensity of condition. As a general guideline a recent European Symposium on PCO recommended a starting dose of 50 mg for every 50 pounds of body weight for the first 3 days, enough to saturate the body tissues, then the amount can be reduced to 1/2 that amount.

CASE HISTORIES

Beverly J., Dallas, Texas

I have been taking Grape Seed Extract for 2 months now. The brown spots on my skin are clearing up, the arthritic lumps on my fingers have gone down, and my gums are more firm. The dentist was concerned about the pockets around my back teeth and was amazed at my last visit when this condition had disappeared. I feel wonderful. I'll never stop taking it.

Tim B., Scottsdale, Arizona

Grape Seed Extract is awesome! I suffer from seasonal allergies and in the past have tried over-the-counter antihistamines which caused me to feel mentally dull and drowsy all the time. After taking the Grape Seed Extract for three days, my allergies cleared up completely without causing any drowsiness. Now I have a clear head and a clear mind. Thanks!

C. M., Scottsdale, Arizona

I was amazed by how fast the Grape Seed Extract cured my hemorrhoids. Within two days they were completely gone and so was the itching and discomfort. Thanks a million!

Christine P., Los Angeles, California

I used to be embarrassed to wear a two-piece bathing suit because of a surgical scar on my abdomen. But since I have been taking Grape Seed Extract over the last two months, the scar has shrunk and now is only faintly visible. Thanks! This means more to me than you can imagine.

Shirley M., Dallas, Texas

A place appeared on my upper arm. It looked red, angry, and precancerous. After two weeks of normal dosage of Grape Seed Extract, it disappeared. My feet do not ache any more either, even wearing high heel shoes.

Peggy G., Scottsdale, Arizona

I was already feeling good when I started taking Grape Seed Extract. I was taking it for its preventive benefits. However, to my surprise, within a few weeks everyone at my work was asking me what I was using on my skin because it looked younger and healthier. I love it.

John G., Scottsdale, Arizona

My Naturopathic Doctor originally prescribed Grape Seed Extract for my jumpy legs, which were keeping me awake at night. In just a few days the jumpiness had completely resolved and I was sleeping great. Three weeks later my Opthamologist told me that I no longer had Glaucoma. The elevated pressure in my eyes was gone.

Robert F., Newton, Iowa

I have had rheumatoid arthritis for fifteen years. My hands had become deformed and crippled. I was taking Prednisone, Methotrexate, Salsalate and Tagamet (to counter the side effects of Salsalate). In spite of all of the heavy drugs I was taking, I was still in constant pain and had no strength in my hands. Within twenty-four hours of starting the Grape Seed Extract, my pain went away completely for the first time in fifteen years. The strength in my hands increased, as did my range of motion and flexibility. I was able to use scissors for the first time in more than a decade. The Grape Seed Extract worked so well that I was able to reduce the drugs.

Larry N., Dallas, Texas

Since running my first Iron Man Triathlon in Hawaii, I developed a lot of joint pains. I thought I would never be able to compete again. But since taking Grape Seed Extract, my joints no longer bother me. Now I'm again training for the next Iron Man.

Diane G., Garland, Texas

For years I suffered with severe psoriatic arthritis. I was taking10 mg of Methotrexate and 175 mg Indocin daily and I was still in severe pain. I could barely walk due to the arthritis, and the psoriasis was raised, red and very itchy. I have had psoriasis for twelve years and nothing had really helped. When I heard of Grape Seed Extract, I decided to give it a try. I began taking 150 mg three times per day. Within 24 hours my pain and stiffness was so much better that I stopped taking the Indocin and haven't taken any since then. After only three days on Grape Seed

Extract, I was able to walk without pain for the first time in literally years. The psoriasis, which used to be unbearable, is no longer raised, itchy or red. And my night vision, which had deteriorated to the point that I was afraid to drive, even improved. Now I can see at night again. For me Grape Seed Extract is simply a miracle.

Bill G., Franklin, Texas

Grape Seed Extract basically gave my life back to me a few months ago when I was very ill with extremely high cholesterol over 400 and triglycerides over 700. I started taking 300 mg Grape Seed Extract per day and continued limiting my fat and sugar intake. Within two months my cholesterol was down to 202 and my triglycerides to 78.

Ryan N., Idaho

Ryan has been diagnosed with extreme allergies, eczema, and asthma. Usually, the skin on his hands is cracked and bleeding around every finger nail and crease. Within two weeks of taking Grape Seed Extract, his hands cleared up completely. His confidence has also improved. He's like a different person.

Darlene H., Dallas, Texas

Recently, my thumbs became so sore that I was really handicapped. I could not button my blouses or skirts, curl my hair, or push the toothpaste out of the bottle. Then a miracle happened. After seven days on the Grape Seed Extract, I had no more pain or discomfort in my thumbs, no discomfort in my knees as I go up stairs, and I have more energy than I thought possible. I am really excited to add that my varicose veins are going away, the brown spots on the back of my hands are disappearing, the nightly itching of the skin on my back has completely gone away, and my legs are very seldom restless at night.

Del S., Salinas, California

I have tried various PCO products and found Grape Seed Extract to be the best. I have diabetes which led to poor circulation in my legs. I developed spider veins in both ankles and my feet became numb and icy cold. Since using Grape Seed Extract, the spider veins and numbness went away completely and my feet are now warm for the first time in three years. I'm feeling great and have been able to cut my insulin intake by fifty percent.

CHAPTER FOUR

4

Glucosamine

The Arthritis Nutrient

INTRODUCTION

Jason had been the athletic type, but no longer. That was before a string of sports injuries had damaged the cartilage in his joints and left him with two bum knees and a bad elbow. The diagnosis: osteoarthritis—a crippling, painful, usually permanent condition. When several surgeries failed to fix the problem, Jason almost gave up hope that he would ever be active again. "I was doing everything that medicine said I should, and it wasn't enough," he says. After a year of taking high doses of anti-inflammatory pain medications, he decided that he had to find another solution.

In his search to learn everything he could about osteoarthritis (OA), Jason discovered that a promising treatment for OA had been used in parts of Europe and Asia for decades. The treatment involves supplementing the diet with an inexpensive nutrient called glucosamine. Glucosamine is a substance which occurs naturally in the body and is necessary for building the cartilage which cushions the joints. Anxious to become active again, Jason dug up research dating back to 1959. The largest of these studies had 1,208 participants who took glucosamine daily. Ninety-five percent of them reported that pain was reduced and mobility increased, with no significant side-effects, and with a continuing benefit 6 to 12 weeks after they stopped the supplement.[1] In another study, microscopic examination of the cartilage before and after treatment showed it had been at least partly repaired.[2] And, in yet another experiment, glucosamine was compared with a commonly prescribed anti-inflammatory pain medicine. By the end of the study, those receiving glucosamine experienced significantly greater mobility and freedom from pain than those receiving the pain medicine.[3] The

1 Tapadinhas, M.J., Rivera, I.C., and Bignamini, A.A. "Oral Glucosamine Sulphate in the Management of Arthrosis: Report on a Multi-Centre Open Investigation in Portugal." *Pharmatherapeutica* 3(3):157-168, 1982.

2 Dovanti, A., Bignamini, A.A., and Rovati, A.L. "Therapeutic Activity of Oral Glucosamine Sulphate in Osteoarthrosis: A Placebo-Controlled Double-Blind Investigation." *Clinical Therapeutics* 3(4):266-272, 1980.

3 Vaz, A.L. "Double-Blind Clinical Evaluation of the Relative Efficacy of Ibuprofen and Glucosamine Sulphate in the Management of Osteoarthrosis of the Knee in Out-Patients." *Current Medical Research and Opinion* 8(3):145-149, 1982.

results of these studies have been duplicated in other significant research over the last two decades.[4, 5, 6, 7, 8]

Jason found the research compelling, as was the fact that European physicians use glucosamine to treat OA, so he began taking the supplement himself. Within two weeks of starting on glucosamine, Jason felt significantly better. Later clinical examination showed that his damaged cartilage was actually repairing itself. Now he says, "I'm back to being a real jock."

But that's not the end of the story. You see, the patient in this story is also a doctor—Jason Theodosakis, M.D. In fact, he's a respected and well-known physician and lecturer in preventive medicine who has trained extensively in exercise physiology and sports medicine. Dr. Theo, as he likes to be called, is also the director of the Preventive Medicine Training Program at the University of Arizona College of Medicine in Tucson.

After his personal success with this "new" OA treatment, Dr. Theo began giving glucosamine to his patients. "The results have been impressive," he says. "I've helped hundreds of people either eliminate the need for surgery or greatly reduce the effects of osteoarthritis." He calls the treatment "the most overlooked medical miracle in America today." His message to OA victims is "There's no reason to suffer any more."

Other respected physicians are beginning to use glucosamine as a part of their OA treatments as well. Andrew Weil, M.D., the best-selling medical author, says "Happily, this seems to be one case where a health fad may actually merit all the attention it's receiving."

Dr. Amal Das, an orthopedic surgeon, has been recommending glucosamine to his patients for three years. "If more people start taking these supplements, it's going to cut down on my business," he says. "I'm having to do less surgery."

Dr. Joseph Houpt, a rheumatologist at the University of Toronto, learned that some of his patients were taking glucosamine on their own. "Enough of them have come back feeling better that I feel it's worth doing a study," he says. He is currently conducting research on 100 patients in his practice.

The mainstream media is beginning to report on glucosamine as well. For example, Newsweek says "...unlike many arthritis fads, this one has some science behind it," and "...if half the people now lining up for the stuff respond to it, arthritis treatment will never be the same."[9]

---

4 Muller-Fasbender, H., et al. "Glucosamine Sulfate Compared to Ibuprofen in Osteoarthritis of the Knee." *Osteoarthritis and Cartilage* 2:61-69, 1994.

5 Noack, W., et al. "Glucosamine Sulfate in Osteoarthritis of the Knee." *Osteoarthritis and Cartilage* 2:51-59, 1994.

6 Pujalte, J.M., Llavore, E.P., and Ylescupidez, F.R. "Double-Blind Clinical Evaluation of Oral Glucosamine Sulphate in the Basic Treatment of Osteoarthrosis." *Current Medical Research and Opinion* 7(2):110-114, 1980.

7 Vajaradul, Y. "Double-Blind Clinical Evaluation of Intra-Articular Glucosamine in Outpatients with Gonarthrosis." *Clinical Therapeutics* 3(5):260, 1980.

8 Crolle, G., and D'Este, E. "Glucosamine Sulphate for the Management of Arthrosis: A Controlled Clinical Investigation." *Current Medical Research and Opinion* 7(2):104-109, 1980.

9 "The Arthritis Cure?" *Newsweek*, Feb. 17, 1997: 54.

OSTEOARTHRITIS FACTS

Approximately 16 million people in the U.S. have osteoarthritis, a painful condition also known as degenerative joint disease. It is the most common form of arthritis, mostly affecting middle-aged and older people. Osteoarthritis is characterized by pain and loss of movement in the hands and weight-bearing joints, such as the knees, hips, feet, and back. What's alarming about OA is the fact that most people over sixty show to have it on X-ray, but may not have actual symptoms yet, according to the Arthritis Foundation.[10]

Currently, the standard treatment for OA involves the use of anti-inflammatory pain medications which only mask the symptoms and do nothing to correct the underlying cause. In fact, regular use of pain killers may actually accelerate the degeneration of cartilage, making the problem worse.[11] When taken regularly, common pain medications have significant side effects like gastrointestinal bleeding and kidney or liver damage.

By contrast, glucosamine has no significant known side effects. It does not mask the pain, it works to help repair damaged cartilage—the root of the problem. In other words, glucosamine relieves pain by helping to restore and normalize joint function. Most people begin to notice a difference in about two to six weeks after beginning to take glucosamine. Then they are able to wean themselves off the pain medicines.

DOCTOR RECOMMENDED?

Is glucosamine the universally recommended treatment for OA here in America? Not yet, but this is quickly changing. There is an extensive body of clinical research proving that glucosamine is an effective OA treatment in both humans and animals. But most of the research has been done in other countries, and doctors here are slow to accept medical advances from abroad.

Why haven't there been American studies? It all boils down to money. Since glucosamine is a nutritional supplement, it cannot be given patent protection as with new drugs. Consequently, there is very little incentive for drug companies to fund research or promote glucosamine by flooding doctors offices with free samples.

However, some American studies are currently in progress. Results from several studies are being analyzed at the Harrington Arthritis Research Center in Phoenix, according to Dr. Louis Lippielo, the center's senior scientist and biochemist. "I think it's pretty promising," he says. "I'd call it the most promising thing in the last twenty years." But for now, you may have to search to find a doctor who is familiar with glucosamine and has read the research. Or you may want to give your doctor a copy of this book and ask him to read the research articles which are listed here.

---

10 The Arthritis Foundation. *Osteoarthritis Fact Sheet,* 1997.

11 Hodgkinson, R., and Woolf, D. "A Five-Year Clinical Trial of Indomethacin in Osteoarthritis of the Hip Joint." *ACTA Orthop. Scand.* 50:169, 1979.

WHICH GLUCOSAMINE IS BEST?

There are several different types of glucosamine. The two most common are glucosamine HCL and glucosamine sulfate. After they are metabolized, both supply the body with the same active ingredient—glucosamine. However, glucosamine HCL is purer, more stabile, and delivers more of the beneficial glucosamine than the sulfate version. And glucosamine HCL has the added benefit of being less expensive, especially when you account for concentration.

Quality is a big issue as well. A University of Maryland analysis found that some brands contained significantly less glucosamine than was stated on the label. So, for best results, buy from a source you know and trust.

CHAPTER FIVE

5

Is Your Home a Healthy Home?

How common household chemicals may gradually be making you and your family sick.

by John K. Beaulieu

IS YOUR HOME A HEALTHY HOME?

It's alarming but true—scientists and doctors have discovered that there is a connection between our health and the use of common everyday household chemicals. If yours is the typical home, you probably use dozens of cleaning and personal care products, purchased at the local grocery store, which contain chemical ingredients that could be harmful to your health and the health of your loved ones.

Since World War II, there has been a dramatic rise in the number of man-made chemicals we use in our homes. The typical home now contains over sixty-three hazardous products that together contain hundreds of different chemicals.[1] At the same time there has been an equally dramatic rise in the incidence of certain chronic health problems. Research indicates that it is more than coincidence that the dramatic rise in these various diseases has coincided with the increased use of hazardous, man-made chemicals in the home.

HAVE WE ALWAYS BEEN THIS SICK?

Around the turn of the century the cancer incidence rate was about one in fifty. Today, one in three Americans will suffer with cancer, with that number expected to reach one in two early in the next century. Cancer is the number two killer of adults and the leading cause of death from disease in children.[2]

---

1 World Resources Institute, *The 1994 Information Please Environmental Almanac* (Houghton-Mifflin, 1994).
2 Paula DiPerna, *Environmental Hazards to Children* (Public Affairs Pamphlets, 1981).

The incidence of central nervous system disorders like Alzheimer's and Multiple Sclerosis increases annually.

Birth defects are on the rise as well. Over 150,000 babies are born with defects each year for reasons unknown. Another 500,000 babies are miscarried early in pregnancy each year with an additional 24,000 miscarried late in pregnancy or stillborn.[3] Infertility is increasing and widespread with over 2 million couples who want children and are unable to conceive.[4]

Asthma was also once a very rare disease. Now the condition is extremely common. The asthma rate has tripled in the last twenty years with nearly 20 to 30 million Americans currently afflicted.[5]

Attention Deficit Disorder in adults and children is rising. In 1993, 2 million children took the drug Ritalin so they could sit still long enough to learn. In 1995, that figure doubled to approximately 4 million, and is expected to reach 8 million by the year 2000.[6]

You or someone you know has probably been touched in some way by one of these illnesses. What could be causing these, and other health problems, to rise and afflict so many otherwise healthy people? Although other factors are involved, more and more scientists are linking these ailments to long-term chemical exposure. And, for most of us, our greatest exposure to chemicals is right in our own homes! We breathe chemical vapors from household products in the air; we absorb chemicals into our skin while using household products to clean our homes or make our bodies clean and smell good; and we swallow small amounts of chemicals when we gargle, or when we eat food from dishes that have been cleaned with chemicals and still contain a thin residue. The home is also where over 1.5 million young children are poisoned each year, and most of the time they are poisoned by a cleaning or personal care product![7]

WHY I WROTE THIS ARTICLE

I realize that you are probably not aware of the potential health hazards present in many household cleaners and personal care products. Unfortunately, most people are not. It is for you that I have written this article. I am not a chemist or a doctor, and I am not trying to promote myself as an expert on household chemicals. However, I have done considerable research on this subject because I want to provide the safest, healthiest home I possibly can for my own wife and children. What I learned is so convincing that I feel I must share it with you and others as best I can.

In this article, you will find quite a bit of information on the connection between household chemicals and your health. I have tried to provide

3 H. Needleman & P. Landrigan, *Raising Children Toxic Free* (Farrar, Straus, & Giroux, 1994).
4 Doris Rapp, *Is This Your Child's World?* (Bantam Books, 1996).
5 Mary Ellen Fise, *Indoor Air Quality* (Consumer Federation of America, 1997).
6 Doris Rapp, *Is This Your Child's World?*
7 The National Safe Kids Campaign, *Poisoning* (1996).

information from the most credible and objective sources possible. You may find the information shocking and very disturbing, as I did. But I want you to know that I do not mean to frighten you. I simply want you to be informed so that you can make a simple, rational decision concerning your health and the health of your loved ones.

THIS ARTICLE HAS A HAPPY ENDING

Happily, there is a simple solution to the problem presented in this article. Some conscientious companies now offer household products that are safer and more natural. Most of these people-friendly and environmentally sensitive products work just as well or better than grocery store brands, and in many cases, actually cost less. So, there's really no reason to risk your health, or the health of your loved ones any longer.

Is your home a healthy home? Right now, it's probably not as healthy as it could be. Read on to learn more.

THEY WOULDN'T SELL IT IF IT WASN'T SAFE . . . WOULD THEY?

When we pick up a product at the local grocery store, most of us like to think we are getting something that has been tested and proven to be safe. After all, we have laws to protect our health and safety, don't we? Actually, the government has very limited power to regulate manufacturers, or require testing of their products. Here are some disturbing facts:

- A product that *kills* 50% of lab animals through ingestion or inhalation can still receive the federal regulatory designation "non-toxic."[8]
- Of the 17,000 chemicals that appear in common household products, only 30% have been adequately tested for their negative effects on our health; less than 10% have been tested for their effect on the nervous system; and nothing is known about the combined effects of these chemicals when mixed within our bodies.[9]
- No law requires manufacturers to list the exact ingredients on the package label.[10]

"Personal care product" refers to just about anything we use to clean our bodies or make ourselves look or smell good. The closest thing to a regulatory agency for the personal care industry is the Food and Drug Administration (FDA), and their power is extremely limited. Here are more unsettling facts regarding personal care products:

- The FDA cannot regulate a personal care product until after it is released into the marketplace.
- Neither personal care products nor their ingredients are reviewed or approved before they are sold to the public.

---

8 Doris Rapp, *Is This Your Child's World?*
9 World Resources Institute, *The 1994 Information Please Environmental Almanac.*
10 Debra Lynn Dadd, *Home Safe Home* (Tarcher-Putnam, 1997).

- The FDA cannot require companies to do safety testing on their personal care products before they are sold to the public.
- The FDA cannot require recalls of harmful personal care products from the marketplace.[11]
- The National Institute of Occupational Safety and Health (NIOSH) analyzed 2,983 chemicals used in personal care products. The results were as follows:

884 of the chemicals were toxic
314 caused biological mutation
218 caused reproductive complications
778 caused acute toxicity
148 caused tumors
376 caused skin and eye irritations.[12]

WARNING: YOU CAN'T TRUST WARNING LABELS!

You may think you know what is in a product and its potential harms by reading ingredient and warning labels. Think again. Manufacturers are not required to list the exact ingredients on the label. Also, chemical names are often disguised by using innocuous "trade names." So even if the chemical is listed on the label, you may not recognize it for what it is.

Even if the harsh and dangerous active ingredients are listed on a package, oftentimes the remainder of ingredients are lumped into a category known as "inert" (not active) ingredients. This term may lead you to believe that these chemicals are not toxic or hazardous. In fact, many of the 1,000 different chemicals used as inert ingredients are more harmful than the active ingredients. The Environmental Protection Agency (EPA) does not require manufacturers to identify most inert chemicals, or disclose their potential harmful effects. Even suspected carcinogens (cancer-causing agents) are used as inert ingredients in household products.[13]

Regarding warning labels, one New York study found that 85% of products they examined had incorrect warning labels. Some were labeled poisonous, but weren't; others were poisonous, but not labeled as such; others gave incorrect first aid information.[14] And there are absolutely no warnings on products about possible negative effects of *long-term* exposure. This is unfortunate because most diseases linked to chemical exposure are the result of long-term exposure.

If we don't know what's in it, and we don't know if it can hurt us, how are we supposed to make an intelligent decision about whether or not to bring this product into our home?

---

11 United States Food and Drug Administration, *FDA Authority Over Cosmetics* (Office of Cosmetics Fact Sheet, 1995).
12 Judith Berns, "The Cosmetic Cover-up," *Human Ecologist* 43 (Fall 1989).
13 John Harte, *Toxics A to Z* (University of California Press, 1991).
14 Debra Lynn Dadd, *Home Safe Home*.

WHY AREN'T MANUFACTURERS REQUIRED TO TEST THESE CHEMICALS?

As we've already discussed, the government has very limited power to regulate manufacturers or require testing of their products. The reason has to do with economics and politics. It takes dozens of years and hundreds of thousands of dollars to fully test *one* chemical. If the government were to require every manufacturer to test every product and prove that it is safe, many manufacturers would be forced to go out of business, and our products would cost about twice as much as they currently do. Besides, who do you think they would test these chemicals on anyway? That's right—animals.

All this would cause a lose-lose situation for politicians. Manufacturers would be angry at them for imposing the expensive testing. And the public would be angry at them for requiring manufacturers to torture and kill all those animals, and for driving the prices of household products through the roof!

Even if a chemical *has* been tested and found to be harmful, you still may not get the truth from a manufacturer. Just look how long it took the tobacco industry to finally admit cigarettes are addictive and cause cancer. Do not wait for any company to spend hundreds of thousands of dollars to confirm that their product definitely causes cancer. Let's exercise our rights as informed consumers and choose manufacturers who make products with safer, more natural ingredients.

WHICH PRODUCTS? WHICH CHEMICALS?

Chemicals that can cause death, cancer, central nervous system (CNS) disorders, learning disorders, birth defects, respiratory illness, and many other health problems appear in most of the cleaning and personal care products in your home. It may be difficult, however, to tell which health risks a particular product poses. Since manufacturers do not list long-term health effects on the packages and are not required to list the ingredients, it's impossible to learn all the health risks by reading the label.

That's why I have provided a short list of product types and general comments about possible health risks below. Of course, every product is different. Even the same product's ingredients can vary from batch to batch depending on the cost and availability of certain chemicals. The following lists of cleaning supplies and personal care products are by no means exhaustive. The possible health effects do not apply to every single brand. However, based on examination of many grocery store brands, chemicals in the following products cause the listed health problems:

CLEANING PRODUCTS

- Air freshener - toxic; may cause cancer; irritates nose, throat, and lungs.
- Disinfectant - very toxic; causes skin, throat, and lung burns; causes coma.
- Drain cleaner - toxic; causes skin burns; causes liver and kidney damage.
- Oven cleaner - toxic; causes skin, throat, and lung burns.

- Window cleaner - toxic; causes CNS disorders; causes liver and kidney disorders.
- Floor/Furniture Polish - toxic; causes CNS disorders; may cause lung cancer.
- Spot remover - toxic; may cause cancer; causes liver damage.
- All-purpose cleaner - causes eye damage; irritates nose, throat, and lungs.
- Toilet bowl cleaner - very toxic; causes skin, nose, throat, and lung burns.
- Chlorinated scouring powder - toxic; highly irritating to nose, throat, and lungs.
- Dishwasher detergent - toxic; causes eye injuries, damage to mucous membranes, and throat.
- Dishwashing liquid - harmful if swallowed; irritates the skin.
- Carpet shampoo - toxic; may cause cancer; causes CNS and liver damage.
- Laundry detergent - toxic; irritates the skin and lungs.
- Bleach - toxic by swallowing; vapors are harmful; causes CNS disorders.
- Stain remover - toxic; may cause cancer; vapors can be fatal.
- Fabric softener - toxic; may cause cancer; causes CNS disorders; causes liver damage.

PERSONAL CARE PRODUCTS

- Shampoo - may cause cancer; irritates eyes, skin, and lungs.
- Dandruff shampoo - may cause cancer; causes organ degeneration; causes CNS disorders.
- Deodorant soap - may cause cancer; causes asthma; irritates lungs.
- Bubble bath - causes bladder and kidney infections; irritates skin and nose.
- Mousse and hair spray - may cause cancer; causes lung disease; irritates eyes and skin.
- Mouthwash - toxic to children; may cause cancer.
- Breath Spray - may cause cancer.
- Cosmetics - may cause cancer; causes CNS damage; irritates skin and lungs.
- Perfume/Cologne - toxic; may cause cancer; irritates skin and lungs.[15,16,17]

ONE COMMON INGREDIENT

Although it would take a second book to cover all the ingredients commonly used in the products above, I want to let you know about one, formaldehyde, as an example. Formaldehyde is used frequently in both cleaning and personal care products because it is a cheap preservative.

The following information is taken from a Material Safety Data Sheet (MSDS) which, by law, must be supplied to anyone who uses any chemical product in the workplace. The MSDS for formaldehyde warns: "Suspected carcinogen; May be fatal if inhaled, swallowed, or absorbed through skin; causes burns; inhalation can

15 Debra Lynn Dadd, *Home Safe Home.*
16 John Harte, *Toxics A to Z.*
17 Ruth Winter, *A Consumer's Dictionary of Household, Yard and Office Chemicals* (Crown, 1992).

cause spasms, edema (fluid buildup) of the larynx and bronchi, and chemical pneumonitis; extremely destructive to tissue of the mucous membrane."[18]

All these symptoms and more are caused by formaldehyde. Yet manufacturers can put formaldehyde in shampoo and not list it as an ingredient![19] You will be shocked to learn that formaldehyde is a common ingredient in baby shampoo, bubble bath, deodorants, perfume, cologne, hair dye, mouthwash, toothpaste, hair spray, and many other personal care items.

Before I go any further, I want to state that the amount of formaldehyde in many of these products is slight. Brushing your teeth every day probably will not give you cancer, but the risk is still there. After all, formaldehyde is still a suspected carcinogen, and if all cancers start from the abnormal growth of one cell, then why allow any amount into or onto your body?

BEWARE OF AEROSOLS

Both cleaning and personal care products come in aerosol cans. I want to warn you of the dangers of aerosols in your home. First, they send a fine mist of toxic chemicals into the air that is easily inhaled and absorbed. Second, this fine mist settles, leaving a coating of toxins on surfaces where children crawl and play and adults eat and sleep. Finally, many of the propellants used in aerosol cans are toxic themselves. Vinyl chloride, one of the most common, can cause dizziness, lack of coordination, headaches, blurred vision, nausea, and death.[20]

I read of a young man named Stuart who became dizzy and collapsed while spray painting bookshelves in his basement. When his wife found him a few hours later, he was dead.

These chemical propellants are also highly flammable. A woman named Laurie received disfiguring burns when the hair spray she was using was ignited by her cigarette. Each year 5,000 people receive emergency room treatment for aerosol-related injuries.[21]

Jimmy, 8, used a hammer and nail to puncture an old aerosol can. The can exploded, hurling pieces of metal into his face and upper chest, cutting him severely.[22]

When you weigh the short-term and long-term harms of aerosol products, I think the smart conclusion is simply to get rid of them.

TOXIC CHEMICALS AND THE HUMAN BODY

Your body is a very complex, very fragile system of chemical reactions and electrical impulses. When you consider a single cell breathes, uses energy, and releases waste much like your whole body does, you can begin to understand how

---

18 Material Safety Data Sheet - *Formaldehyde.*
19 Debra Lynn Dadd, *Home Safe Home.*
20 John Harte, *Toxics A to Z.*
21 Dr. Ted Ferry, *Home Safety Desk Reference* (Career Press, 1994).
22 Dr. Ted Ferry, *Home Safety Desk Reference.*

even small amounts of harmful chemicals can affect the performance of the body's processes. Chemicals enter the human body in three ways: ingestion, inhalation, and absorption.

INGESTION

Ingestion brings to mind the image of a young child opening the cabinet under the sink and drinking something deadly. Well, each year nearly 1.5 million accidental ingestions of poisons are reported to U.S. Poison Control Centers. The majority of the victims are under the age of twelve and have swallowed a cleaning or personal care product.[23] It amazes me how many deadly chemicals are stored under sinks or on bathroom counters and bathtubs within easy reach of young children.

INHALATION

It may surprise you to learn that poisoning by inhalation is more common, and can be much more harmful, than ingestion. When something harmful is swallowed, the stomach actually begins breaking down and neutralizing the poison before it is absorbed into the bloodstream. However, when you inhale toxic fumes, the poisons go directly into the bloodstream and quickly travel to organs like the brain, heart, liver, and kidneys.

Many products give off toxic vapors which can irritate your eyes, nose, throat and lungs, and give you headaches, muscle aches, and sinus infections. This process of releasing vapors into the air is called *outgassing*. Outgassing occurs even when a chemical is tightly sealed in its container. If you doubt this, simply walk down the cleaning aisle at your local grocery store and notice how strongly it smells of toxic vapors even though all the containers are sealed tight.

ABSORPTION

Finally, you need to realize the potential threat absorption poses. One square centimeter of your skin, an area less than the size of a dime, contains 3 million cells, four yards of nerves, one yard of blood vessels, and one hundred sweat glands.[24] We've all heard the ads for nicotine patches and analgesic creams. These medicines work by being absorbed into the bloodstream through the skin. Even some heart medicines are administered through transdermal (through the skin) patches.

Any chemical that touches the skin can be absorbed and spread throughout the body. This can even happen when you come in contact with a surface that was treated with a chemical days, or even weeks earlier. I had no idea that my children could be harmed by crawling across the kitchen floor my wife had just cleaned. I thought we were being conscientious, not reckless. Since we no longer have products which contain harmful chemicals in our home, I no longer worry when

23 The National Safe Kids Campaign, *Poisoning*.
24 Nancy Sokol Green, *Poisoning Our Children* (The Noble Press, 1991).

I see my baby daughter crawling across the floor or putting her fingers in her mouth. I know she is not absorbing or ingesting toxic residues.

HOME IS WHERE THE CHEMICALS ARE

Home is where you are most likely to be exposed to toxic chemicals. After all, you spend 80 to 90% of your time indoors, most of that at home.[25] This fact is important when you understand that in one five-year study, the EPA found that airborne chemical levels in homes were as much as seventy times higher inside than outside.

When toxic household chemicals release vapors into the air, they have nowhere to go. During the oil shortages of the 1970s, builders began making houses as energy efficient as possible. The result has been homes that keep toxic indoor air tightly sealed inside.

Exposure to toxic indoor air may have a devastating effect on your health. One fifteen-year study found that women who worked at home had a 54% higher death rate from cancer than women who had jobs outside the home.[26] The study concluded that the increased death rate was due to daily exposure to the hazardous chemicals found in ordinary products. Some experts argue that 30% of all cancers stem from exposure to toxic chemicals.[27]

Not all of the health effects are fatal, however. According to a special legislative committee of the Commonwealth of Massachusetts, 50% of all health problems are caused, in part, by deteriorated indoor air quality.[28] A hangover is the side-effect of non-lethal ethanol poisoning (getting drunk). How many days do you wake feeling "hung over," with aches and pains or nausea? Perhaps the air in your home is poisoning you. How many bottles of pain-killers have you purchased to rid yourself of headaches, possibly brought on by your fabric softener?

The good news is that by switching to safer, more natural products, you can rid yourself of these symptoms altogether. You can make your home a healthy home.

IMMEDIATE EFFECTS OF CHEMICAL EXPOSURE

Could this happen in your home? When Peter Schwabb of Seattle, Washington, was a year old, he crawled over to the dishwasher to watch his mother unloading it. Suddenly, he put a finger into the detergent dispensing cup and ate a fingerful of wet but undissolved Electrasol. In minutes his face was red and blistered, and the inside of his mouth and his tongue were burned white. Because of a series of lucky circumstances, Peter was in the hospital within minutes and he recovered in a few days.

While Peter was in the hospital, there was a little girl across the hall who (according to Peter's mother) ate some dishwashing detergent and required seven operations to reopen her scarred esophagus.[29]

---

25 World Resources Institute, *The 1994 Information Please Environmental Almanac.*
26 Nancy Sokol Green, *Poisoning Our Children.*
27 John Harte, *Toxics A to Z.*
28 Doris Rapp, *Is This Your Child's World?*
29 Shirley Camper Soman, *Let's Stop Destroying Our Children* (Hawthorn Books, 1974).

Another 18-month-old boy had to eat through tubes for five months and at last count has had thirty operations. Detergent is what destroyed his throat, too.[30]

Three-year-old Jason Whitely, of Tulsa, Oklahoma, died a lingering and horrible death two weeks after swallowing three ounces of a hair rinse containing ammonia.

Seven-month-old Adrian Gonzalez, Jr., of Belen, New Mexico, crawled through a puddle of spilled bleach, which gave him third-degree burns on 50% of his tiny body and burned his lungs from the fumes as well. It took him four days to die.[31]

The real tragedy here is that all of these accidents could have been prevented. A simple decision to use safer products could have meant that these children would not have had to suffer and die. Unfortunately, most parents don't realize that they have a choice.

MORE DANGEROUS THAN GUNS

It may shock you to learn that according to the National Safety Council, more children under the age of four die of accidental poisonings at home than are accidentally killed with guns at home.[32] Among children age five and under, the most common poison is a cleaner or personal care product.[33]

Ninety percent of all poisonings occur at home between the hours of 4 and 10 PM, when children are home from school and playing in the house.[34] Young children are especially vulnerable. They learn by putting things in their mouths. This is even more frightening when you consider the number of products that look like something else. Window cleaner looks like blueberry drink. Ammonia looks like apple juice. Many poisons come in bright, colorful containers with small, obscure warning labels that young children can't read. Remember the skull and crossbones symbol? It's a symbol that children can identify easily, but manufacturers are no longer required to display it on most household products.

Lennon Miller, 18 months, of Memphis, Tennessee, drank lemon-scented furniture polish, enticed no doubt by the attractive smell. He lived during a day of suffering, and died in John Gaston Hospital of chemically-induced pneumonia.[35]

ACCIDENTS HAPPEN TO ADULTS, TOO

Young children are not the only ones at risk for chemical injury. Poisoning is the number one accidental killer in the home, accounting for over 3,000 deaths in 1985 and over 4,000 deaths in 1990. These chemicals are also responsible for thousands of injuries each year.[36]

A 34-year-old man received burns on his arm after using a caustic drain-

30 Shirley Camper Soman, *Let's Stop Destroying Our Children.*
31 Shirley Camper Soman, *Let's Stop Destroying Our Children.*
32 *Accident Facts* (National Safety Council, 1993).
33 The National Safe Kids Campaign, *Poisoning.*
34 The National Safe Kids Campaign, *Poisoning.*
35 Shirley Camper Soman, *Let's Stop Destroying Our Children.*
36 Home Safety, *USA Today* (February 13, 1997).

cleaner in his bathroom sink. Fifteen minutes after applying the chemical, he ran water into the sink, but the remaining residue splashed on his arm.[37]

A woman poured boiling water into a can of oven cleaner, according to the directions on the can. As she carried the can from the table to the oven, it spilled, burning her hand and producing large quantities of ammonia gas, which gave her a choking cough.[38]

But most of the health problems related to chemicals in the home are not because of accidents like these. Most chemical-related health problems are the result of exposure to toxics day after day, year after year.

LONG-TERM EFFECTS OF CHEMICAL EXPOSURE

Before I begin discussing the long-term effects of exposure to toxic chemicals in cleaning and personal care products, I want to make two points that I think are very important. First, the different diseases and conditions linked to chemical exposure are usually the result of *long-term* exposure. Just as one cigarette is not likely to give you cancer, one non-acute exposure to chemicals in cleaners probably won't harm you either. But we're talking about cumulative exposure to many different products: your mouthwash, conditioner, cologne or perfume, laundry detergent, window cleaner, and so on. When you consider all the products and all the chemicals you come across each day, you can begin to understand the potential for long-term harm.

Remember, the long-term effects of exposure to most chemicals in household products are not known. And nothing is known about what happens when they mix within our bodies. Drinking alcohol while using certain drugs can be a deadly combination. Could other chemicals mix in our bodies in a similarly fatal way?

My second point concerns your body. What most doctors and scientists who investigate and treat chemical-related illness contend is that the *amount* of chemical a person is exposed to is not as important as *how sensitive* a person might be.[39] Some people can drink three beers and not be intoxicated. Others can feel groggy after drinking less than one beer. It all depends on a person's size and weight and the strength of their detox system. The same concept applies to chemical exposure.

YOUR DETOX SYSTEM

Your body has a system that destroys and eliminates toxins. After all, many things that appear naturally in the environment are toxic, and we need to have a strong defense system against them. Organs like the kidneys and liver filter out and remove toxins. Our blood contains T-cells that attack foreign agents. However, many people have overloaded or very weak detox systems. High levels

---

37 Dr. Ted Ferry, *Home Safety Desk Reference.*
38 Dr. Ted Ferry, *Home Safety Desk Reference.*
39 Dr. Doris Rapp, Is *This Your Child's World?*

of toxins and a poor nutritional state leave many people more susceptible to the effects of chronic chemical exposure.

Even healthy people can be affected. When exposed to a certain toxin, the body will respond by producing more of the enzymes needed to destroy the poison. In a sense, the body has "masked" the poisoning.[40] It has prevented the effects of the poisoning from being felt, even if the effects would have been mild. But, this has stressed the immune system, possibly leaving a person vulnerable to infection.

By switching to cleaners and personal care products that are not full of toxins, you can reduce the stress on your detox system, possibly leading to a healthier life. I have not missed a day of work due to illness in over two years. I have not seen a doctor for illness in three years. My children have been to the doctor for illness only twice in three years. I believe this is, in part, the result of my wife and me deciding to switch to safer and more natural products. I encourage you to do the same. It's one decision your family can live with.

BIRTH DEFECTS

Birth defects are the leading cause of death among children ages one to four. According to the March of Dimes, one in twelve children is born with a congenital defect. Environmental factors, including exposure to toxic chemicals, cause 7 to 11% of these defects. Sixty percent of birth defects have unknown causes. Toxic chemicals are suspected in these cases as well.[41]

In fact, the Council on Environmental Quality's report on chemical hazards to human reproduction concluded that, "the relationship between exposure to chemicals and human reproductive impairment may be an important area of public health concern that deserves more scientific investigation."[42]

Birth defects have been found in a number of animal species where high levels of toxic chemicals are present. A 1996 University of Minnesota study found higher rates of birth defects in children who lived in areas of the state where agricultural chemicals were used the most.[43]

Dr. Marion Moses of the Environmental Sciences Laboratory at Mount Sinai Medical Center in New York strongly recommends that, as far as toxins and carcinogens are concerned, the unborn child should have NO exposure; and where there is doubt about any chemical, err on the side of the child and prevent as much exposure as possible. "If we wait until we have absolute proof for all agents, it may be too late for the child," Dr. Moses stresses.[44]

Thalidomide is a tragic example of a substance that was touted as safe by its manufacturer but was later proven to cause horrible birth defects. Children whose mothers took the drug were born with deformed limbs or no limbs at all.

---

40 Nancy Sokol Green, *Poisoning Our Children.*
41 Paula DiPerna, *Environmental Hazards to Children.*
42 Paula DiPerna, *Environmental Hazards to Children.*
43 *Dioxins* (National Wildlife Federation Office of Conservation Programs, 1997).
44 Paula DiPerna, *Environmental Hazards to Children.*

This tragedy destroyed the belief that the placenta was a complete barrier between the baby and the environment. It also served as a wake-up call to how chemicals within the body can disrupt normal fetal development.

The NIOSH study I mentioned earlier stated 314 chemicals that appear in personal care products can cause biological mutations.[45] Many of these chemicals, including known carcinogens, can reach the unborn child.

Chemicals can also cause defects by damaging the egg cells in women. All the eggs a woman will ever have are produced while she is still a baby in the womb. By the fifth month of fetal life, the 3 to 4 million eggs a woman is born with have localized in her ovaries. Chemical exposure at any point can destroy or damage these cells, leaving her infertile or prone to birth defects or miscarriage.[46] Once damage has occurred, repair is almost impossible.

In men, exposure to chemicals can affect sperm development profoundly. A study of male Vietnam veterans found they were 70% more likely to have a child with a birth defect due to chemical exposure.[47] Many of the same chemicals are now found in products used every day around the home.

The presence of solvents in drinking water has been linked to leukemia and birth defects in California, Massachusetts, and New Jersey.[48] You may be exposed to a number of potentially harmful solvents every day, including ethanol, styrene, trichloroethylene, vinyl chloride, diethylene glycol, and toluene. All of these appear in common household products.

INFERTILITY AND MISCARRIAGE

More than 2 million American couples who want to have children are unable to do so. Perhaps you or someone close to you is living with this heartache. It may surprise you to learn that between 1938 and 1991 the sperm count of males in industrialized countries has decreased 50% in quantity and quality. A cross-sectional study of college men found that 25% were sterile. Projected figures place the male sterility rate at over 50% early in the next century.[49]

Women's fertility has also been negatively affected by the increased use of chemicals. In 1934, only twenty-one cases of endometriosis existed in the entire world. Now there are over 5 million women with this condition, which causes infertility, in the United States alone.[50] High levels of toxins have been found in German women with endometriosis. Female monkeys exposed to dioxins had an increased rate of this condition also.[51] Combine the decreased sperm count with the prevalence of endometriosis and you can see just how the infertility rate could grow so large and affect so many.

---

45 Judith Burns, "The Cosmetic Cover-up".
46 H. Needleman & P. Landrigan, *Raising Children Toxic Free.*
47 Dr. Doris Rapp, *Is This Your Child's World?*
48 Ruth Winter, *A Consumer's Dictionary of Household, Yard and Office Chemicals.*
49 Dr. Doris Rapp, *Is This Your Child's World?*
50 Dr. Doris Rapp, *Is This Your Child's World?*
51 Dr. Doris Rapp, *Is This Your Child's World?*

Even women who can conceive are experiencing extremely high rates of miscarriage. In 1988, more than 600,000 women experienced a miscarriage, and in most cases the cause was unclear.[52] In many cases a woman's body will reject an unborn baby if it detects a profound defect of some kind. We may begin wondering if we are living in a time when more babies have defects. Or perhaps the chemicals that enter the body somehow send mixed or wrong messages.

Many chemicals, including alkylphenol, found in many industrial and household detergents, are known hormone disrupters. This means they act like hormones and can actually change behavior, mood, development and any other bodily functions regulated by hormones. It concerns me that the delicate balance of chemicals our bodies naturally produce and need to function properly can be skewed by synthetic, toxic chemicals.

CANCER

No word strikes more fear into people's hearts than "cancer." Although the death rate from cancer has declined, the incidence rate has not. Cancer rates continue to grow in almost every segment of the American public. Breast cancer and prostate cancers have doubled in the past fifty years. Testicular cancer has tripled during the same period. Over 550,000 people will die of cancer during this year.[53]

The majority of cancer cases are due to environmental factors.[54] Most experts agree that as many as 80 to 90% of all cancers can be avoided by making certain lifestyle changes. Please understand that "environmental factors" include everything in the environment, including diet, sleep patterns, etc. Some experts argue that 30% of all cancers are caused by exposure to toxic chemicals.[55]

The National Cancer Institute has a list of twenty known carcinogens and over 2,200 chemicals that are probable carcinogens.[56] Many of these chemicals are in the cleaners and personal care products you buy at your local grocery store. The National Toxicology Program is urging that fifteen more chemicals be added to the list of known carcinogens, including an organic solvent used in grease-cutting cleaners.[57]

Cancer tumors start from the mutated growth of one cell. Even minimal exposure over a long period of time can put you at risk of developing cancer. The risk may not be that great, but for me there is no acceptable level of risk when it comes to cancer. I know I can't completely eliminate all potential hazards from my life, but I no longer put myself at risk for cancer by exposing myself to the unregulated, dangerous chemicals that appear in products like laundry detergent, bathroom cleaner, hair conditioner, and cologne.

---

52 H. Needleman & P. Landrigan, *Raising Children Toxic Free.*
53 *National Cancer Statistics Review 1973-1994* (National Cancer Institute, 1997).
54 John Harte, *Toxics A to Z.*
55 John Harte, *Toxics A to Z.*
56 World Resources Institute, *The 1994 Information Please Environmental Almanac.*
57 *Press Release* (National Institute of Health, May 2, 1997).

CANCER IN CHILDREN

I know my children are safer, too. Each year 6,500 children in the United States are diagnosed with cancer. Cancer remains the leading cause of death from disease for children over the age of five, accounting for over 2,100 deaths a year.[58]

The tragedy is that only 20% of cases of childhood cancer are due to genetic factors. Remember, we now know that carcinogens can cross the placental barrier. Exposure to carcinogens in the womb may cause childhood cancer by causing tumor development or by altering the baby's genes, leaving them with a predisposition to cancer. Dr. Robert Miller of the National Cancer Institute states that many carcinogens have a short enough latent period that exposure in the womb could lead to the diagnosis of tumors in the pediatric age period.[59]

Finally, I think it is important to remember that current cancer rates reflect past toxic exposure. Only time will tell what the legacy of our increased use of household products full of toxic chemicals will be.

ASTHMA

The American Lung Association now estimates that 3.7 million American children and 20 million adults presently have asthma. That is three times more victims than just twenty years ago.[60] Once again, environmental factors are under strong suspicion. I have already told you that most Americans spend 80 to 90% of their time in air-tight buildings, most with less than adequate ventilation. One study concluded that the majority of the 400,000 annual emergency room visits for severe asthma attacks are brought on by poor indoor air quality. Each year, asthma claims the lives of over 4,000 people and costs Americans over 6 billion dollars in medical costs and lost time from work and school.[61]

Doctors know that irritation of the lungs by chemicals can trigger asthma attacks. Long-term exposure to chemicals can contribute to the development of asthma. This is especially true with children. A child's immune system is not fully developed until she is twelve years old. A one-year-old has practically no detox system at all.[62]

Out of germ-phobia, some parents constantly spray disinfectant into the air and on all surfaces in their baby's nursery. What they may not realize is they are exposing their children to formaldehyde, cresol, phenol, ammonia, ethanol, and chlorine. It takes much less of these chemicals to harm a baby than an adult. Babies' bodies are much smaller and they breathe at ten times the rate of adults. The average child visits the doctor twenty-three times in the first four years of life, with the most common complaint being respiratory ailment.[63] When babies get sick, the last thing they need is to have irritating chemicals filling their lungs.

58 H. Needleman & P. Landrigan, *Raising Children Toxic Free.*
59 Paula DiPerna, *Environmental Hazards to Children.*
60 Dr. Doris Rapp, *Is This Your Child's World?*
61 Mary Ellen Fise, *Indoor Air Quality.*
62 Paula DiPerna, *Environmental Hazards to Children.*
63 National Center For Health Statistics, 1997.

CNS DISORDERS

Central Nervous System (CNS) disorders can range from headaches and dizziness to Multiple Sclerosis, Parkinson's Disease, and Alzheimer's Disease. We know that many chemicals that appear in our household products are neurotoxins. Some act as depressants, some as stimulants, and some cause mood swings. Others act similar to alcohol, leaving a person lethargic, unable to concentrate, and with a loss of balance.

It's important, once again, to remind you that only 10% of the chemicals that appear in household products have been tested for negative effects on the nervous system.[64] And we know nothing about the long-term effects of exposure to these chemicals.

We do know that young people are destroying their brains by abusing aerosol products and inhaling their deadly fumes. In fact, aerosols are the drug of choice for many of these people. This is very frightening.

Doctors have also identified a condition known as toxic encephalopathy, brought on by repeated exposure to solvents over several years. Symptoms include memory loss, behavioral changes, emotional instability, confusion, inability to concentrate, neurological and personality changes, and problems with manual dexterity.[65] Chemicals that cause this condition are in household products. They include chlorinated hydrocarbons, aromatic hydrocarbons and aliphatic hydrocarbons. You need to remember that the amount of chemicals a person is exposed to is not as important as the strength of a person's detox system. Extremely small amounts of chemicals can have severe effects on certain individuals.

Alzheimer's Disease receives so much attention because it is so prevalent and yet remains such a mystery. Around 4 million people currently suffer with Alzheimer's.[66] Although we have known about this disease for some time, recently the number of cases has grown dramatically. Approximately 14 million people will have the disease by early in the next century, and it may surpass cancer and stroke numbers as a cause of death.[67]

Although there seems to be a genetic link to the cause of Alzheimer's, scientists admit it is too weak to explain the prevalence of the disease. Most research points to environmental factors. Aluminum, a known neurotoxin, is the number one suspect. However, researchers are looking at other toxins and their possible link to this horrible disease. Hopefully, science will find the answers.

Not every CNS problem is as dramatic as Alzheimer's, but some can be almost as debilitating. Betty J., of Albuquerque, New Mexico, suffered from severe migraine headaches for years with major attacks occurring every six to eight weeks. Unfortunately, the medication she was taking was as disabling as the

64 Dr. Doris Rapp, *Is This Your Child's World?*
65 N. Ashford & C. Miller, *Chemical Exposures, Low Levels and High Stakes* (Van Nostrand Reinhold, 1991).
66 Dr. Doris Rapp, *Is This Your Child's World?*
67 Dr. Doris Rapp, *Is This Your Child's World?*

headaches. She would spend a week to ten days in bed until the migraines finally passed and the medication wore off. As you can imagine, this caused great hardship for her, especially with regard to her work.

After doing a little investigation, Betty decided to rid her home of toxic chemicals. She threw out everything she had purchased at the grocery store and used only natural, environmentally sensitive products. Her life changed dramatically. She no longer needed to take painkillers to get out of bed and the recurring migraine attacks stopped.

Disbelieving her own success, Betty purchased a bottle of bleach to see if chemicals were indeed the cause of her problem. Within minutes of opening the bottle, she had another migraine headache. Betty became a true believer in the need to rid your home of toxic, chemical-laden cleaners.

ATTENTION DEFICIT DISORDER AND OTHER LEARNING DISORDERS

By the year 2000, 8 million children in America will be taking Ritalin so they can sit still long enough to learn to read and write.[68] Ritalin is a "Class-2" narcotic. What could be wrong? Why do we need such a powerful drug to help control our children's behavior? Most veteran teachers will tell you that the increased use of Ritalin is not the result of an increased awareness in ADD, as some would argue, but an increase in the actual number of cases. Think back to when you were in school. Was half of your class out of control? Were most of your friends taking medication for hyperactivity? Again, we must find out just what is wrong!

The problem is that many young people are being misdiagnosed. According to Doris Rapp, M.D., an expert on the treatment of environmental illness, as many as two-thirds of the millions of children on Ritalin are actually suffering from acute allergic reactions to environmental agents. Removal of certain chemicals or a profound change in diet could solve the problem.[69] These children do not need powerful drugs.

Young people are exposed to so many chemicals that many of them develop sensitivities. This happens because their detox system burns out even before it fully develops. Then they become susceptible to the effects of even traces of chemicals. I want to state one more time that when it comes to toxins, the amount of exposure is not as important as how sensitive a person is. Children need much less exposure than adults do to develop negative symptoms.

CHEMICAL VAPORS IN SCHOOLS

Take the case of Ryan. When he was four, he began going to school. He would leave feeling fine, but come home feeling weak and tired, clinging tightly to his mother. While in the gym at his school, he became so weak that he had to be carried out. Ryan's mother noticed that they sprayed the table tops and rest area of his classroom with a popular aerosol disinfectant.

---

68 Dr. Doris Rapp, *Is This Your Child's World?*
69 Dr. Doris Rapp, *Is This Your Child's World?*

Ryan's doctor, an environmental specialist, tested Ryan. She sprayed a four inch area of a paper towel with the same disinfectant and placed it a few feet away from Ryan. Within thirty minutes, Ryan was obviously different. He could no longer hold his pencil and his writing skills completely collapsed. Several tests confirmed his reaction.[70] William, another eight-year-old boy, had a similar reaction when exposed to chlorine fumes.[71]

Ryan's reaction might be considered severe, but it represents a growing number of young people who are reacting to chemicals in the air in their homes and school. I wonder how many children experience learning problems because of chemicals in the environment. Even if the number is only slight, it is unacceptable. We should try to remove any possible impediment from our children's future, and that begins with providing the healthiest home possible.

Eight-year-old Peter's first class in the morning was taught by a teacher who smoked heavily and smelled strongly of perfume. In this class, arithmetic, Peter typically had difficulty remembering, thinking, and completing his work. His teacher noticed on some days he could not even add two and two.

Peter improved over the course of the morning when he had another teacher who did not smell of either tobacco or perfume. However, the smell of perfume from lunchroom aides and the odor of cleaners from the dish room caused his ability to learn and concentrate to deteriorate again.

Peter's doctor confirmed his sensitivities to many chemicals. Perfumes, colognes, and fragrances can contain harmful chemicals such as formaldehyde, toluene, ethanol, acetone, methyl chloride and benzene derivatives. All can damage the nervous system. Peter now goes to school with an oxygen tank in case he has a severe reaction.[72]

Eleven-year-old Warren always did well in school. His grades were in the 90th percentile. Exposure to phenol caused him to develop multiple ear infections and led to a progressive decline in his grades. After several tests, Warren's doctor confirmed his sensitivity to phenol. Warren eventually transferred schools to escape exposure during the day. Fortunately, his grades returned to normal.[73]

According to Sherry Rogers, M.D., also an environmental specialist, the symptoms produced by chemical sensitivity are as varied as the people affected.[74] While children like Peter and Warren might react with a breakdown of learning ability, children like Chuck become hyperactive. When Chuck was six years old, he would make very loud noises, become uncontrollably bouncy, and hit other children when exposed to certain chemicals. Fumes from furniture polish affected him so strongly that he told his mother he wanted to jump off the roof![75]

---

70 Dr. Doris Rapp, *Is This Your Child's World?*
71 Dr. Doris Rapp, *Is This Your Child's World?*
72 Dr. Doris Rapp, *Is This Your Child's World?*
73 Dr. Doris Rapp, *Is This Your Child's World?*
74 Sherry Rogers, *Chemical Sensitivity* (Keats Publishing, Inc., 1995).
75 Dr. Doris Rapp, *Is This Your Child's World?*

These stories hardly reflect the array of reactions that children who are chemically sensitive exhibit. Reaction is unpredictable and can change in time. The bottom line is, you *can* protect your children. You can limit, if not eliminate, their exposure to neurotoxins. By switching to brands that do not use chemicals like phenol and formaldehyde, you can help them reach their full potential.

MULTIPLE CHEMICAL SENSITIVITY

Multiple Chemical Sensitivity (MCS), or Environmental Illness (EI), are the names for an assortment of problems that can affect any part of the human body. Chemicals found in cleaners, personal care products, food, plastics, and even water, can cause this condition. Persons suffering with MCS lack the ability to adequately detoxify their bodies. Symptoms include: headaches, severe fatigue, hyperactivity, muscle pain, joint pain, stomach and bowel problems, constant congestion, muscle twitches, and asthma-type symptoms. Other symptoms include emotional and behavioral problems, depression, loss of memory, and inability to learn or concentrate. More and more people are coming forth, reporting these symptoms, and having their sensitivities confirmed.[76,77]

I have read the accounts of many victims, and personally spoken with dozens more. Most were very sensitive to chemicals in cleaning and personal care products. They had debilitating body aches, headaches, depression and other nervous disorders. Thankfully, the majority I have talked to received nearly complete relief by switching to people-friendly household products.

Dr. William Rea, a world-known environmental doctor in Dallas, Texas, reports that of all the patients he has seen with MCS, only 13% report developing the condition after a one-time acute poisoning. Sixty percent report developing the condition as the result of long-term slow poisonings involving minimal amounts of toxins. Only 28% of the cases he has documented are work-related. A staggering 72% of the cases are people who have been exposed to chemicals at home or at other places.[78]

Dr. Rea sites the following factors as influencing the onset of MCS:

- Total Toxic Body Burden - This is the sum of all toxins in the body. When the accumulation overloads a person's detox system, MCS can occur.
- Nutritional State - The more nutrient-depleted a person's body is, the more likely they are to develop MCS.
- Synergisms - This means the combination of the different chemicals in the body will have a stronger effect than individual toxins.
- Bioaccumulation of Toxins - This refers to how less dense tissues, like fat cells, can actually absorb and accumulate chemicals. Without the time and nutrition for the body to cleanse itself, the accumulation level can be dangerous.[79]

76 William J. Rea, *Chemical Sensitivities* (1997).
77 Sherry Rogers, *Chemical Sensitivity.*
78 William J. Rea, *Chemical Sensitivities.*
79 William J. Rea, *Chemical Sensitivities.*

According to Doris Rapp, M.D., Multiple Chemical Sensitivity is common. Most physicians who practice environmental medicine, including herself, estimate that 25 to 50% of today's population is sensitive to one degree or another.[80]

Nancy, a young, vibrant, well-trained teacher, developed MCS over a period of eight years. She became fatigued, experienced muscle aches, constant ear ringing, difficulty concentrating, blackouts, and severe depression. She became so sensitive that even the nuance of chemical odor made her ill. Scents in her body lotions, make-up and hair spray made her so confused that she could not tell time or recall the names of her students. A whiff of perfume caused her to laugh uncontrollably and twitch.

During a leave of absence, she was too tired to get out of bed, take a shower, or prepare a snack. Her condition was traced to, among many things, phenol in the disinfectants used in the bathroom near her classroom. After two years of therapy, she began to feel better, but she still carries a charcoal filter mask everywhere she goes and fears a total relapse.[81]

Sister Martha, a dedicated teacher, was assigned by her school to tutor students who needed extra help. Unfortunately, the only available room was a converted custodial closet located between two bathrooms. The vapors from cleaners, disinfectants and deodorizers from the bathrooms constantly filtered into this room through vents in the walls.

After tutoring for awhile in this room, Sister Martha developed a persistent, nagging cough, joint stiffness and swelling, facial spasms, excessive mucus, and vision problems. She was able to find a doctor who began to treat her sensitivities. Even after extensive treatment, she still lives with many limitations. Although she has eliminated toxins in her home, she cannot remain in a public place like a mall for more than a few minutes. She still needs to take an anti-allergy extract and can drink only purified water.[82]

Both of these stories represent extreme cases of MCS. Most people who suffer with MCS do not have such profound symptoms, but rather experience symptoms like recurring headaches, muscle aches, depression, and chronic fatigue.

Hopefully, more will be learned about MCS and treatments will improve. However, I think the focus should be on prevention. By reducing the amount of toxins in your home, you can help to reduce the risk for MCS in a loved one.

SOME FINAL THOUGHTS

As I am finishing this article, I have just learned that the FDA has proposed a ban on phenolphthalein, a phenol derivative found in laxatives that has been linked to cancer in laboratory animals.[83] I believe that many more chemicals will be banned as we learn about the long-term effects of exposure. Other phenol

80 Dr. Doris Rapp, Is This Your Child's World?
81 Dr. Doris Rapp, Is This Your Child's World?
82 Dr. Doris Rapp, Is This Your Child's World?
83 HHS News (U.S. Department of Health and Human Services, August 29, 1997).

derivatives still appear in many personal care and cleaning products. I strongly urge you not to expose yourself to any chemical that could possibly cause cancer.

At the same time, another company is pulling their tire cleaning product off the shelves because even a tiny amount of the product can kill a child. This product was marketed in a spray bottle! I don't have to tell you parents how children love those spray bottles.

I understand that life is full of risk. When you drive on the highway, there is risk. Going outside in a thunderstorm is risky. It is important to distinguish between what are avoidable risks and what are unavoidable risks. Many Americans have quit smoking, changed their diet, and started exercising because they want to reduce their risk for heart disease, cancer, and a host of other possible conditions. They avoid placing themselves at risk.

In the same way, I encourage you to make your home a healthy home by eliminating toxic chemicals. By removing the dangerous cleaners and personal care products, you remove the potential harms they cause. You eliminate the unnecessary risk for cancer, ADD, nervous disorders, asthma, birth defects, MCS, infertility, and a host of other problems.

I said at the beginning of this article that there is a happy ending —a solution to this problem. Conscientious manufacturers offer people-friendly products at great prices that are just as, if not more effective than hazardous store brands. Talk to the person who cared enough to share this article with you. I am sure they will know where you can get these products.

I am glad you took the time to read this article. I pray that it has opened your eyes to a menace you may not have been aware of before. I hope you now are able to make an informed choice about what you bring into your home.

And may your home be a healthy home.

CHAPTER SIX

6

Healthy Body

The following section provides self-help guidelines for common health conditions. These recommendations are based on medical research and the clinical experiences of health care professionals. However, please note the following disclaimer:

> ***It is recommended that you develop a good relationship with a physician knowledgeable in the art and science of natural and preventive medicine. The information in this book is not a substitute for the care you should be receiving from your primary physician. In all cases involving a physical or medical complaint, please consult your physician.***

ABDOMINAL DISTRESS

The area between the pelvis and the rib cage contains more organs and more sites for discomfort than any other area of the body. Colic or upset stomach in infants, indigestion, reactions to foods, and constipation are common problems that can occur. The bowel, liver, pancreas, kidneys, spleen, stomach, and gallbladder are all possible sites of distress.

Of all abdominal distress, gas and indigestion account for 80% of complaints. Abdominal distress is often caused by unhealthy eating habits. While we should all drink at least eight glasses of pure water a day, this water should be consumed between meals rather than at meal time. When we drink too many liquids with our meal, digestive enzymes are diluted. This, in turn, can be manifested as indigestion or abdominal pain caused by bloating and gas.

Upon feeling discomfort in the abdomen, one should try to remember if food was ingested which was of questionable freshness. The so-called *summer flu*, which many experience, is actually due to bacterial toxicity from improperly handled food.

Overeating in the evening hours, or eating in a hurry, packs food in the stomach before nerve and hormone stimulation can properly begin the digestive process. Eating rich, fatty meals stresses the stomach, gallbladder, and pancreas, which slows down digestion and allows ever-present bacteria to begin fermentation and putrefaction in the bowel.

Constipation is at epidemic levels in our country. Eating high roughage foods helps hold moisture in the bowel, giving the muscles of the bowel physical material to propel along its some 26 feet. This roughage rapidly carries ingested toxins, proliferating bacteria, and metabolic byproducts out of the body. Experts agree that 20 to 30 grams of fiber per day is advisable for adults. As a result of a mechanized and refined food lifestyle, the average American eats 7.3 grams of fiber each day.

Suggested Treatment: Celebrate eating. Give thanks. Eat as many meals with soft music and candlelight, in the presence of people you love, as possible. Drink adequate amounts of liquid including 2 or 3 cups of *G'Day Melaleuca Tea* each day—between meals. Slow down! Use *This is Fiber?!* bars to supplement your daily intake of roughage. Each bar supplies 7 grams of the much-needed fiber! Get 20 to 40 minutes of moderate daily exercise to promote circulation within the abdomen and stimulate bowel peristalsis. Multiple small meals are generally preferable to one or two large meals each day. Take *The Vitality Pak* and *Cell-Wise* daily to encourage proper metabolism and waste excretion from cells. If indigestion occurs, use *Calmicid* as directed. *Calmicid* provides fast relief of acid indigestion, heartburn, and gas. It aids digestion with ginger root and helps relieve cramping with chamomile and fennel seed.

To correct colic in infants, give several teaspoons of warm *G'Day Melaleuca Tea* during the day and before bed. Many infants have also found relief when given *ProVex* once or twice daily. Simply open a capsule and dissolve the *ProVex* in distilled water, juice, or expressed breast milk.

ABRASIONS

These injuries occur when your skin slides across coarse materials, such as concrete, gravel, or asphalt. The top layers of skin are damaged, causing nerves, blood vessels, and lymph vessels to be exposed to the air. This causes immediate pain and creates an opportunity for germs to enter the body. After the bleeding and oozing stops, a dry protective scab will usually form within a few hours and is nature's protection against infection.

Suggested Treatment: Washing the area gently, yet thoroughly, with *Antibacterial Liquid Soap* and cool water quickly reduces the pain. (Warm or hot water increases nerve stimulation and pain in most people.) Allow the stream of water to wash off all visible particulates. Pick out any embedded material. Apply *Triple Antibiotic Ointment* or *Mela-Gel* and allow to remain open to the air if possible. Otherwise, use a loose bandage saturated with *Triple Antibiotic Ointment* or *Mela-Gel* to prevent sticking. Repeat administration of *Triple Antibiotic Ointment* or *Mela-Gel* as frequently as needed for several days until the wound is adequately covered with a scab.

ABSCESSES

These painful, pus-filled sacks of infection can occur in or on any surface of the body. Abscesses may start from a cut, scratch, pimple, ingrown hair, ingrown fingernail or toenail, hemorrhoid, or pierced ears for earrings. Occasionally the lack of proper treatment of an infection can produce a characteristic swollen, red, painful lump. The typical bacteria which causes abscesses is *Staph. epidermis* which is found on healthy skin. While antibiotics are often necessary, the overuse of antibiotics, both by prescription and in the meat we eat, has led to the development of many antibiotic-resistant strains of bacteria.

Suggested Treatment: Begin drinking *G'Day Melaleuca Tea* in place of other liquids 3 to 4 times each day. Apply *T36-C5* to the abscess. To encourage drainage and drive the *T36-C5* into the wound, apply hot moist packs over the area. If the abscess can be lanced and drained, soak afterward in solution of 1 oz *Sol-U-Mel* and 2 Tbs. of Epsom salts in 1 quart of warm water. If the area is unable to be soaked, saturate a hand towel in the solution, wring it out, heat in a microwave for 1 minute then apply to the affected area for 10 minutes. Repeat every hour to speed draining. Apply *Triple Antibiotic Ointment* or *Mela-Gel*. If needed, cover with gauze to absorb any seeping fluid and keep the area clean.

ACHES AND PAINS (MUSCLE)

see Muscle Strain

ACNE

Overproduction of the oil glands in the skin can dry and harden, forming blackheads. These may produce a local bacterial infection and pimples. Acne is common to those working in hostile chemical environments, people suffering with hormonal imbalances, or those under physical or emotional stress. Skin blemishes in individuals of all ages arise from improper nutrition, toxicity, and rapidly changing needs for hormonal regulation. Familial or lifestyle traits are learned from our parents and often give the appearance of a genetic link.

Suggested Treatment: Suspect food allergies and experiment with elimination diets or get tested by a natural physician. Minimize sugar. Drink 3 to 4 cups of *G'Day Melaleuca Tea*, hot or iced each day, in addition to the regular 8 glasses of pure water you should normally drink. Reduce fats to less than 20% of total calories. Perspire for 20 minutes each day, preferably from exercise, but sauna or steam baths work also.

Shower while washing entire body with *Antibacterial Liquid Soap* or *The Gold Bar* and a soft wash cloth. For those who prefer bathing, always put 1 oz of *Sol-U-Mel* in the tub. Especially avoid eating cooked oils such as margarine and potato chips. Get 20 grams of fiber including a *This is Fiber?!* bar daily. Take *The Vitality Pak* and *Cell-Wise* with every meal for the added nutrient benefits of vitamin A, zinc, B vitamins, and vitamin C.

The *Zap-It! Acne Treatment System* was especially developed for the prevention of acne. Consistent use of this system usually delivers clear skin. Clean skin with *Zap-It! Facial Wash.* Apply *Zap-It! Astringent,* then apply *Zap-It! Pore Clarifying Cream.* Carry *Zap-It! Quick Stick* for convenient treatment away from home.

In addition, you can apply *T36-C5* to any developing pustule. Apply *T36-C5* to blackheads to clear the plugged oil duct. Apply *Moistursil Problem Skin Lotion* afterward to keep moisture in skin and resist oil accumulation. Avoid dry brush or friction rubs with alcohol as this naturally stimulates oil production. Get enough rest.

ADD AND ADHD

see Attention Deficit Disorder

AIR PURIFICATION

The quality of the air you breathe in your home may be robbing you of good health. Modern energy-efficient homes, by virtue of their air-tight design, often trap chemical vapors from furniture, carpets, and building cements, in addition to mold, fungus, yeast, and bacteria from moist condensation in heating and cooling air ducts, soil from house plants, and under sink areas. There is a literal zoo co-inhabiting in our homes. Many respiratory, eye, ear, nose, and throat complaints appear in doctors' waiting rooms because of over-exposure to foul household air. Changes of seasons often shift populations of these microbial species as growing conditions fluctuate

Suggested Treatment: Convert your home to Melaleuca products, replacing toxic cleaning and personal care products with safer Melaleuca products. The outgassing of toxic vapors from both personal care and home hygiene products significantly increases air quality problems.

Remove browning leaves from house plants immediately. Provide good drainage for house plants, and do not over water.

Change furnace and cooling air return filters monthly during extreme weather usage. Spray all filters and vents often with diluted *Sol-U-Mel.* To do a Melaleuca oil purge of your house two to twelve times a year, attach an inverted open bottle of *T36-C5* on the furnace intake filter. The high air volume will diffuse the entire contents of the bottle throughout your house over the next 12 to 36 hours (depending upon temperature and relative humidity). This treated air flows throughout all the rooms and stops the growth of bacteria, molds, fungus and viruses.

Take *ProVex* or *ProVex-Plus* when exposed to toxic substances.

ALLERGIC REACTIONS

Skin rashes, itching skin, sore throat, runny nose, sinus congestion, eye irritation, headaches, and fatigue are common symptoms of allergy sufferers. While individuals vary in their degree of sensitivity to allergic substances, it is important to minimize discomfort and prevent complications such as infections. Many of the aromatic oils from *Melaleuca alternifolia* have local-acting anti-inflammatory and desensitization effects.

Suggested Treatment: Always try to avoid the allergen when possible. Your natural physician can help you determine the substances you are reacting to and begin a program to gain permanent desensitization. Applying *T36-C5* directly to exposed skin reaction sites (hands, arms, legs, feet, scalp, neck, and abdomen area) usually neutralizes the local histamine reaction and reduces symptoms. A word of caution—do not apply any Melaleuca products near or in the eyes. Avoid rubbing the affected skin to prevent further irritation. *Moistursil Problem Skin Lotion* or *Mela-Gel* can be applied afterwards to give long lasting protection. Soaking in a bath containing 1 oz of *Moistursil Bath Oil* (and 1 oz of *Sol-U-Mel* if infections are present) offers an added soothing effect.

Remember, allergies are the result of an unhealthy immune system, so maximizing your nutrition is essential. Besides eating wholesome foods, *Mel-Vita, Cell-Wise,* and *ProVex* or *ProVex-Plus* taken with every meal give extra protection against allergies by providing antioxidants in the form of beta carotene, vitamin C, and vitamin E, citrus bioflavonoids, and proanthocyanidins (antioxidants reduce histamine levels which cause the itching, rashes, and burning). The calcium in *Mela-Cal* often gives immediate relief from sneezing and general body aches during a reaction.

For both chronic and acute allergies/hayfever, many people find relief from *ProVex* or *ProVex-Plus*. These may need to be taken at the rate of 1 capsule for every 25 pounds of body weight per day in order to provide the most relief and/or prevention of allergies.

When your nose and throat are affected by hay fever, dust, pollen, or food reactions, try this: breathe hot steam from either a vaporizer or bowl of steaming water with 10 drops of *T36-C5* and 2 capfuls of *Sol-U-Mel* for a minimum of 15 to 20 minutes twice a day (all night is even better). This gives a welcome relief.

ALOPECIA

see Hair Loss

ANEMIA

Insufficient red blood cells and/or hemoglobin causes fatigue and lack of motivation. *Blood loss* due to hemorrhage somewhere within the body or *decreased production* of red blood cells are the two sources. There are several varied conditions that result in anemia. Iron deficiency due to poor nutrition is most common in teenage girls and the elderly. Heavy menstrual flow is often associated with anemia. Drugs such as aspirin thin the blood and cause micro-hemorrhage in the gastrointestinal tract. This can cause anemia, especially in women who use this medication for menstrual pain and cramps. Copper, zinc, protein, and B vitamins are essential for a healthy supply of red blood cells. Deficiencies of any of these can lead to various types of anemia which are often difficult to diagnose. A sudden drop in red blood cells (hemolytic anemia) or hemoglobin (hypochromic anemia) is one of the early warning signs of cancer. Infestation of bowel parasites from outdoor pets can also lead to anemia and malnutrition. Often, anemias can only be clearly identified by a complete blood chemistry and blood cell study. Your natural physician can provide further information regarding anemias.

Suggested Treatment: Avoid over-the-counter drugs. Ask your doctor about the side effects of any prescription medications. Eat an adequate amount of raw fruit and vegetables, whole grains, and fish. Take *The Vitality Pak, Cell-Wise,* and *ProVex* or *ProVex-Plus* regularly to supplement iron and essential nutrients to insure adequate red blood cell building blocks. Drink 2 cups of *G'Day Melaleuca Tea* each day to maximize kidney detoxification. Get 20 minutes of moderate exercise five times each week to adequately oxygenate the body.

ANGINA

see Chest Pains

ANTISEPTICS

An ounce of prevention is worth a pound of cure when it comes to germs that cause infection. Any break in the skin is a potential site for infection. Use protective gear, clothing, boots, hats, back braces, or goggles when needed.

Suggested Treatment: Bathe or shower with *Antibacterial Liquid Soap* or *The Gold Bar* which leaves a fine layer of Melaleuca oil on the skin. For jobs where your hands will become dirty, use *Clear Defense, Antibacterial Liquid Soap,* or *Sol-U-Mel* as a preventive hand glove. If an injury occurs, there is a barrier between you and the awaiting germs. You can simply rinse the pre-treated area with warm water and lift the germs off with the soap. Apply *Moistursil Problem Skin Lotion* afterward. This is especially good for mechanics to prevent grease and grime (often loaded with germs) from forcing their way into the skin. It is also especially effective around farm machinery and animals.

ANXIETY

When a person gets excited there are several adrenal hormones that are released to combat the stress. Anxiety is a condition when these hormones are either set off randomly or they do not return to normal after stimulation. While adequate exercise and rest are vital, nutritional supplementation can also be beneficial. Menopause or PMS can induce anxiety in some women.

Good nutrition should include *The Vitality Pak* and *Cell-Wise*, along with *ProVex*, *ProVex-Plus*, or *ProVexCV*. *Luminex* and *Sustain* taken as directed can be very helpful. Hormonal fluctuations resulting in anxiety during times of PMS or menopause might improve with *EstrAval* taken daily.

APPENDICITIS

Pain in the lower right abdomen which causes a bent posture and an elevated white blood cell count are sufficient evidence to wheel a person into surgery and remove the appendix—just before it bursts! The human appendix is a lymphatic collector of wastes protecting the valve between the small and large intestine. It's purpose is not clearly known, but it carries a reputation of getting infected and being the cause of many failed human endeavors. Apparently, food and bacteria can lodge in the appendix and breed putrefaction and infection. Constipation commonly precedes appendicitis. See the section on Abdominal Distress.

Suggested Treatment: Prevention is the best solution. Drink 2 to 4 quarts of liquids including water, *G'Day Melaleuca Tea*, and juices each day. Drink hot water upon rising each morning to get the system primed and hydrated. Exercise moderately at least 5 days each week. Get 30 grams of soluble and insoluble fiber each day including *This is Fiber?!* to prevent constipation.

ARMS/LEGS ASLEEP

Loss of feeling in the arms or legs (paraesthesia) can be caused by a temporary pinch of a nerve while sleeping or having someone sit on your lap. It also can be progressive due to peripheral circulatory problems where the sensory nerves in the extremities do not receive enough blood. Some people who have handled toxic solvents, paints, cleaners, pesticides, or herbicides experience extremity paraesthesia soon after.

Suggested Treatment: Use *Pain-A-Trate* on any tender muscles in your neck and upper back. If you are susceptible to paraesthesias, do not try to sleep in a moving vehicle without an inflatable cushion behind your neck. Trade legs often when holding someone on your lap. Be checked by a chiropractor when you have any kind of traumatic accident to your neck or back. Always have adequate ventilation when using volatile solvents or paint. Remember—at first your nose will alert you to the danger. If unheeded, the signal will diminish until you "*get used to it.*" Use only environmentally safe sprays.

ProVex or *ProVex-Plus* should be taken daily. Take *The Vitality Pak* and *Cell-Wise* every few hours to offset the destruction of nutrients by these substances in your liver. Eat *This is Fiber?!* to carry the substances out of your digestive tract quickly. Drink extra water, *G'Day Melaleuca Tea* and

Sustain for maintaining blood sugar during environmentally stressful times. Exercise after an exposure to harsh volatile chemicals to flush the lungs. Sweat from exercise or in a sauna or steam bath to wash out as many toxins as possible.

ARTHRITIS

Hot, red, painful and stiff swollen joints of the hands, wrists, elbows, neck, back, hips, and knees are common symptoms of arthritis. More remedies are sold to treat arthritis than any other common condition. Arthritis can be caused by old injuries, allergies, gout, mineral deficiencies, hyperactive immune response, toxicity, poor circulation, handling of cold things, or prescription drug side effects.

Suggested Treatment: The best long term treatment is the one that gets at the cause. Some cases of arthritis respond to reducing white sugar, white flour, nicotine, caffeine, and alcohol. Generally avoid cold temperatures to the affected joint. For osteoarthritis, take *Replenex Joint Replenishing Complex* to help rebuild cartilage and restore normal joint function. For all forms of arthritis, take *ProVex* or *ProVex-Plus* to help reduce inflammation. Some forms of arthritis respond well to resting the joint, while other forms, such as osteoarthritis, respond to motion such as knitting. *Pain-A-Trate* and *T36-C5* can be applied to the affected area with a heating pad or hot moist pack to achieve rapid relief of pain and stiffness. Taking *The Vitality Pak* and *Cell-Wise* with each meal provides essential trace nutrients for reducing further injury and increasing healing. Since dehydrated joints ache, drink more liquids, including 2 to 4 cups of *G'Day Melaleuca Tea* per day.

ASTHMA

Congestion and restriction of the lungs causes labored breathing and wheezing, and affects one out of every twelve people. Many are small children. Although it is associated with airborne allergies and occasional food sensitivities, improvement can occur by following a few simple suggestions

Suggested Treatment: Identify and restrict all sensitizing substances (see Air Purification). Rid your home of all toxic personal care and home care products. Convert your home to Melaleuca products, beginning with the *Ecosense Laundry System*.

Take *The Vitality Pak* with each meal for adults and *Vita-Bears* with each meal for children, along with *ProVex-Plus*, to increase resistance to attacks. Apply *Pain-A-Trate* to the chest of adults and children before bed. Get enough rest. If congestion exists, increase the amount of *ProVex-Plus* taken until you find the level that provides relief. *ProVex-Plus* and *The Vitality Pak* or *Vita-Bears* have given many asthma sufferers much relief.

Further relief comes from a humidifier or vaporizer with water plus 10 drops of *T36-C5* and 2 capfuls of *Sol-U-Mel*.

Adults can try adding 10 to 20 drops of Tabasco sauce (capsicum) in a few ounces of water and drinking it immediately before a meal to reduce congestion and thin mucous in the lungs.

One drop of *T36-C5* on a cotton tipped swab gently used to clean pollen and dust from each nostril before bed has helped many children.

ATHEROSCLEROSIS

Hardening of the arteries can lead to high blood pressure, shortness of breath, strokes, and cold hands and feet, as well as senility and premature aging. Cholesterol (LDL—the bad kind) and ionic calcium make up part of the *"cement"* which lines arteries of the liver, bowel, lungs, brain, kidneys, legs and arms. Several common-sense suggestions can help.

Suggested Treatment: Begin taking *ProVexCV*, *The Vitality Pak*, and *Cell-Wise* daily! Every adult should be on this regimen for prevention of atherosclerosis.

Stop smoking and avoid smokers. Avoid animal fats and cooked vegetable fats. Reduce total fat to less than 20% of your total diet. Eat a good variety of raw fruit and vegetables each day. Begin a gradual daily exercise program. Eat an *Access Bar* 15 minutes before exercising and drink *Sustain* drink one half hour after exercising to speed up the fat burning process. Drink 3 to 4 cups of *G'Day Melaleuca Tea* daily.

ATHLETE'S FOOT

Public showers offer a great opportunity to contact the fungus that causes *tinea pedis*, known as athlete's foot. Blistering often occurs when the immune system becomes sensitized to the fungus. When the fungus infects the upper body, this is known as *tinea corporis*, or ringworm, causing raised and reddened rashes with clear centers. Long term athlete's foot often involves the toenails and often totally destroys the nail plate and may enter the bone. This infection will persist indefinitely until treatment is effective. The general health of the individual tends to determine the magnitude of the infection and extent of the symptoms.

Suggested Treatment: As in most infections, prevention is the best treatment. Always wear shower sandals when in public showers, such as athletic locker rooms and swimming pools. Spray feet with *Melaleuca Essentials Antibacterial Foot Spray* and apply *Dermatin Antifungal Creme* between toes and to bottoms of feet immediately after showering. *Sole to Soul Revitalizing Foot Scrub* and *Revitalizing Foot Lotion* can also be used to cleanse and stimulate improved circulation. Direct sunlight and air drying the feet after showering or swimming is also a helpful preventive measure. Take *The Vitality Pak, Cell-Wise,* and a *ProVex* product with each meal to optimize trace nutrients. Drink 2 to 3 cups of *G'Day Melaleuca Tea* daily.

To eliminate the athlete's foot, clean the affected area well with *Antibacterial Liquid Soap* and water. (For stubborn infections, clean the affected area by adding 1/2 tsp. *Moistursil Bath Oil* and 1/2 tsp. *Sol-U-Mel* to one-quart warm water and soak feet in this solution for 20 minutes morning and night for one week.) Pat dry. Apply *Dermatin Antifungal Cream* as directed. Or apply *T36-C5*, followed by *Moistursil Problem Skin Lotion* or *Mela-Gel* each morning and night. If there is no improvement after one week, discontinue use and consult your physician.

ATHLETIC INJURIES

The human body is designed for motion. Actually, everyone is an athlete—you are either actively practicing or you are not. More middle-aged and elderly people are enjoying the benefits of regular exercise than ever before. Typical athletic injuries in all ages include pulled muscles, strained ligaments and tendons, bruises and muscle cramps. Of course, proper warm up and cool down and stretching before and after working out are essential, but what can we do to prevent so many injuries? See the sections on Abrasions, Bruises and Cuts in this book.

Suggested Treatment: Athletic injuries typical to all ages include pulled muscles, strained ligaments and tendons, bruises, and muscle cramps. Take *The Vitality Pak* every meal, as well as *ProVex*, *ProVex-Plus*, or *ProVexCV* each day, to optimize tissue strengthening nutrients. Take more *Mela-Cal* if you have muscle cramps after a work out. Eat an *Access Bar* 15 minutes before exercise to inhibit adenosine and open fat stores in the body for energy. *Sustain* drink can be mixed in your water bottle for continual replenishment of waning blood sugar.

Pain-A-Trate should be in the equipment bag of every athlete. Regular application of *T36-C5* stimulates circulation to injured tissue. Immediate application of *Pain-A-Trate* to any closed injury will start the healing process. Ice is good for injured joints, muscles, tendons and ligaments. Apply ice for no more than 5 to 10 minutes at a time. Longer treatment periods can actually cause frostbite or reverse the anti-inflammatory effect. Heat can cause problems so it should be avoided, in most cases, for the first 24 to 48 hours after an injury to bruised or pulled muscles. Chronic or untreated injuries that do not resolve should be seen by a chiropractor or physician trained to treat sports injuries.

ATTENTION DEFICIT DISORDER (ADD AND ADHD)

Attention deficit disorder and attention deficit hyperactive disorder are found in children and adults who have a reduced attention span and variable pattern of behavior problems. Many clinical studies indicate that there is a link with dietary and environmental factors. Food and chemical sensitivities frequently play a role. Areas of the brain appear over-stimulated while others show reduced electrical activity. Simple sugar cravings and intolerance appear to also be indicated. Several studies indicate a link with essential fatty acid deficiencies within the brain.

Suggested Treatment: Identify any and all foods, food additives, household cleaners, and synthetic substances shown to be reactive, and remove them from the child's environment. Convert your home to Melaleuca cleaning and personal care products. Reduce fried foods, cooked and rancid oils (potato chips, french fries, etc), sugar, (including artificial sweeteners), and food colorings. Have a metabolic and nutritional physical exam provided by a certified clinician

The following supplements, along with appropriate dietary changes, may be useful to help improve symptoms: *The Vitality Pak* to help maintain proper nutrition, *Luminex* to maximize cerebral circulation, *ProVex-Plus* to reduce free-radical activity and to help reduce sensitivities to allergens, *Cell-Wise* to help maintain cell structure in the brain, and *Sustain* to help maintain proper blood sugar balance and reduce sugar cravings.

BABY TEETH

All 20 baby teeth are usually present by the age of 4. Children will lose these teeth between the ages of 5 and 12 as the size of the growing head and mouth require larger teeth. Care and protection of these teeth is important to insure a healthy environment for the permanent teeth, which may need to last 75 to 100 years.

Suggested Treatment: Do not put a child to bed with a nursing bottle of fruit juice or formula. This is the most common cause of *"dissolved"* baby teeth and the need for capping. As soon as the baby teeth appear, brush with *Koala Pals Sparkling Tooth Gel* or *Classic Tooth Polish,* after every meal. Give your child *Vita-Bears* to insure strong healthy teeth.

BACK PAIN

More than one half of the adult American population suffers with back pain. Our sedentary lifestyle, motorized transportation, and poor diets cause a large portion of our discomfort. Stretching and strengthening exercises, eating a healthy diet, maintaining our healthy weight, supplementing calcium, magnesium, and micro-nutrients, and correcting spinal injuries before they become chronic can go a long way toward reducing back pain

Suggested Treatment: Apply *Pain-A-Trate* to over-worked muscles. Apply moderate heat (use cold immediately after injury or acute pain 5 to 10 minutes each hour for first 6 to 24 hours before using heat). Use *T36-C5* on skin over spasming back muscles to promote the relaxation reflex. Take *Mela-Cal* every 2 to 4 hours to relax muscles. Drink 2 to 4 cups of *G'Day Melaleuca Tea* each day. Take *ProVex* or *ProVex-Plus* daily, in addition to *The Vitality Pak* and *Cell-Wise,* to help heal collagen structures in your back.

BACTEREMIA

see Boils

BALDNESS

see Hair Loss

BARBER'S ITCH

Caused by a fungus from an improperly cleaned razor, shaving cream brush, or electric shaver, the typical reddened rash is less common since the use of disposable razors and canned shaving foam or gel. See the section on Athlete's Foot in this book.

BATHING

One of the most self-pampering events of life is taking a hot bath. Getting the most out of your time and effort is essential. Showers expose persons with respiratory or skin sensitivities to 8 to 10 times the amount of chlorine as bathing. Chlorine sensitive persons should run hot bath water and allow it to de-gas for about 5 minutes with the window open or the vent fan running before plunging in. Never take long baths (30 minutes or more) with a breeze in the room, as the lungs are susceptible to infections from cool air when the body is heated above 100 degrees. Put *Sol-U-Mel* (1 oz per tub) in the water to thoroughly sanitize and disinfect the skin. The *Moistursil Bath Oil* or the *Hydrotherapy Foaming Bath* are real therapy for the pores of the skin. See the sections on Sauna Baths and Hot Tubs in this book.

BED SORES

Also known as decubitus ulcers, bed sores occur when people are bedfast or confined to a wheel chair. A lamb's wool or *"egg carton"* foam pad can be placed under the person to prevent the deep crater sores from forming. Daily inspection is important to identify the blanched skin heralding the onset of a bedsore. Once started, bed sores can lead to infections and delayed healing. Prevention is the best treatment.

Suggested Treatment: Healing begins at the outer edges and works inward when pressure is removed from the area. Apply *T36-C5* to any blanched skin areas before the sore begins. It can often be halted at this stage. If a sore is present, gently wash the area with a washcloth and *Antibacterial Liquid Soap* enriched with one capful of *Sol-U-Mel* in 1 quart of warm water. Apply *Triple Antibiotic Ointment*. Cover with loose gauze. Use minimum amount of tape. Repeat washing and *Triple Antibiotic Ointment* every 8 hours until the wound heals. This can take from one day to several weeks depending upon the overall health of the individual. NOTE: Bedsores should be taken very seriously in diabetics, persons on immune suppressive drugs, and those with leg ulcers due to poor circulation.

BEE AND WASP STINGS

Bees are territorial creatures. They defend their territory by injecting a powerful chemical, formic acid, into the intruder. This injection also contains traces of immune reactive agents that can provoke violent reactions in humans.

Suggested Treatment: Carefully remove the stinger by scraping it out. Wash the area with *Antibacterial Liquid Soap* and cold water. Immediately apply *T36-C5* or *Mela-Gel* to stop pain and prevent secondary infection. Do not use any other home remedies, such as baking soda, with the Melaleuca products in this treatment. Reapply every 15 minutes until all signs and symptoms are gone. Four to six treatments may be necessary. Take *ProVex* or *ProVex-Plus* immediately and continue for 24 hours.

NOTE: When a person is allergic to bee or wasp stings, this can be life threatening. The allergic person should carry an antidote kit containing adrenaline and benedryl. Administer this according to the directions before any other therapy. Shortness of breath or difficulty breathing, puffy or swollen throat or eyes, rapid heart rate, dizziness, or profuse sweating are signs of allergic reaction and can appear within 10 to 30 minutes after being stung. *DO NOT DELAY; GET EMERGENCY HELP!*

BENIGN PROSTATIC HYPERPLASIA (BPH)

As men age, and especially after "Male Menopause," testosterone is inefficiently utilized in the prostate gland. Physical trauma (sitting), stress, excessive animal fat intake, and nutrient deficiencies induce oxidation of testosterone into dihydrotestosterone. This causes the prostate gland to enlarge and become less functional. Slow or dribbling urination, difficulty starting urination, incomplete emptying of the bladder, getting up multiple times at night, and reduced sexual function accompany this condition. Almost one half of men over the age of 55 experience symptoms of BPH. BPH does not indicate cancer and should be differentiated from this more severe condition.

Suggested Treatment: Get annual prostate exams after age 50 including the sensitive blood tumor marker for prostate cancer called PSA. Prevention is the best treatment. Regular hot baths seem to reduce the incidence of BPH. Native Japanese men have a lower incidence of BPH and other prostate problems due to their custom of very hot baths. Americans tend to shower and have a statistically higher incidence of most prostate problems. The ingredients in *ProstAvan* have a proven effect in helping prevent BPH and should be taken every day by men over the age of 40. One extra tablet for every decade past 40 is advised. *Luminex* is advised to maximize cerebral circulation and hormone regulation. *The Vitality Pak*, *Cell-Wise,* and *ProVex* or *ProVex-Plus* are also vital. Three cups of *G'Day Melaleuca Tea* each day is also helpful.

BLACK EYE

Bruising almost anywhere on the head resulting from an auto accident, reaching for the last cookie (just kidding), or even extensive dental work can cause a black eye.

Suggested Treatment: Apply an ice pack as soon as possible after the injury, to slow down facial swelling. Do not use any Melaleuca products near the eye, as its aromatic vapor is drying to the eye and causes pain. Take *The Vitality Pak* as well as *ProVex* or *ProVex-Plus* to speed healing and prevent easy bruising.

BLACKHEADS

see Acne

BLADDER INFECTIONS

Bladder infections, most often in women, can be bothersome at least, and a potential full-blown illness at worst. Underwear made of synthetic fabric causes excessive perspiration, which leads to bacterial growth at the opening of the urethra. Not drinking enough water encourages bacteria to grow within the urethra and bladder. Repeated infections are a cause for alarm. Note: Recurrent infections treated with antibiotics can lead to highly resistant strains of bacteria.

Suggested Treatment: Drink 2 to 6 cups of *G'Day Melaleuca Tea* along with 2-4 quarts of pure water each day. Wear cotton underwear. Douche with *Nature's Cleanse* weekly to reduce bacteria in the area. Add 1 oz of *Sol-U-Mel* in rinse water of washing cycle when laundering undergarments. Use the *Ecosense Laundry System*.

BLEEDING

Bleeding from an open wound should receive immediate attention. Pulsating bleeding or spraying blood from a wound is an indication of a cut artery. Get trained emergency help immediately.

Suggested Treatment: Apply direct finger or hand pressure to the area, sufficient to stop the bleeding. Elevate the body part above the heart if the bleeding is on an arm or leg. Apply *T36-C5*, *Triple Antibiotic Ointment*, or *Mela-Gel* under a pressure bandage to slow bleeding, to prevent infection, and to prevent the bandage from sticking to the wound. Change dressing every day until healing forms a dense scab. Do not apply *Pain-A-Trate*, as it contains natural aspirin which can prevent blood from clotting naturally.

BLEEDING GUMS

Deep plaque or periodontal infections can cause bleeding gums, swollen gums or dental pain. Brushing too hard is a common cause. Chronic vitamin C deficiency, alveolar (jaw) bone loss, or chemical poisoning are other possible causes. The mouth is the literal window to overall health of the body!

Suggested Treatment: Switching to Melaleuca dental care products often gives relief from bleeding gums. Regular brushing with *Classic Tooth Polish* and rinsing with *Breath-Away Mouthwash* is a good way to control the buildup of bacteria-causing plaque. Daily flossing with *Exceed* and chewing *Insta-Fresh* gum can clean between teeth where a brush cannot reach. Drinking 2 to 4 cups of *G'Day Melaleuca Tea* per day helps promote a healthy environment in the mouth. Take *The Vitality Pak*, *Cell-Wise*, and *ProVex* or *ProVex-Plus* while eating a healthy diet. Get professional dental care if bleeding, pain, or swelling of gums persists.

BLISTERS

Friction, chemical, or heat injuries can cause blistering which may lead to blood poisoning if not properly treated.

Suggested Treatment: Do not puncture blisters. They can easily become infected. Mother Nature's bandage is the best. Immediately apply *T36-C5* to a developing blister. Ice is often helpful also. This will usually prevent further development. If the blister has formed, apply *Pain-A-Trate*, *Mela-Gel* or *Triple Antibiotic Ointment* and a cushioned bandage. The fluid pressure should reduce within 6 to 12 hours. Repeat treatment daily until the overlying skin sags, breaks open on its own, and is replaced by a non-sensitive layer of skin from below. Continue treatment as long as there is pain, swelling, or redness.

BODY LICE

Seeing a louse on a piece of clothing is one thing; seeing it on yourself or a friend is something else. Melaleuca oil products are a safe alternative to the prescription drug lindane, as testified by many of you.

Lice infestation (*Pediculosis*) involves the head (*P. capitus*), the trunk or extremities (*P. corporis*), or the genital area (*P. pubis*). Originally, body lice prefer birds and almost any hairy mammal other than man. They will settle for second best (humans) when a warm puppy or chicken is absent, but will selectively crawl to these animals if given a choice. The louse lives directly off of blood after biting and puncturing the skin, hence it can easily spread a multitude of diseases. It lives in hairy areas including eyebrows, eyelashes, or beards, where it lays its grayish-white eggs (nits) which can be seen with a magnifying glass on the hair follicles. The eggs hatch in three to fourteen days where the sluggish, overweight-looking insects seem eager for their first meal. Multiple families of lice cause excruciating pain, irritation, and itching. They are transmitted by contact with objects such as combs, hats, and shared garments. For this reason it is common among school children.

Suggested Treatment: Immediately upon suspecting or seeing evidence of lice, shampoo with *Natural Shampoo* and bathe in a mixture of 1 oz of *Sol-U-Mel* and 1 oz of *Moistursil Bath Oil*. Afterward, massage *T36-C5* into scalp and hair to soften and dislodge nits. Don't be stingy with the oil! Comb the oil through the hair. To fumigate the live insects, wrap your hair in a hot moist towel for 10 minutes. Repeat every second day for at least 5 treatments (10 days). Avoid re-infection. Wash all clothing and bedding with *MelaPower* laundry detergent, 1 capful *Sol-U-Mel*, and hot water.

BODY ODOR

Bacteria, yeast, bowel putrefaction, dental disease, vaginitis, chronic tonsillitis, kidney or liver failure, as well as a number of chronic degenerative disorders and chemical exposures, can lead to a foul body odor. Perfume was invented in Europe during the Dark Ages when the prevailing theory was that bathing and exposing the body to the air was the cause of infectious disease. WRONG! However, it may prevent people from getting close enough to you to give you a disease. Foul-smelling sweat (bromhyperhidrosis) is observed in some diabetics, nervous individuals, chronic smokers, and persons on certain prescription medications. People who have a bad odor become desensitized to it and need to be told by someone who cares. Read the sections on Bathing, Sauna Bath, and Yeast Infections in this book.

Suggested Treatment: Drink 2 to 4 cups of *G'Day Melaleuca Tea* each day for detoxification. Take *The Vitality Pak* regularly. Brush regularly with *Classic Tooth Polish* or *Fluoride Tooth Gel,* floss with *Exceed*, and use *Breath-Away Mouthwash* after meals. Use *Hot/Cool Shot Mouth Spray* before going out in public, and chew *Insta-Fresh* gum frequently. If you are a smoker, STOP! Bathe instead of shower. Use *Antibacterial Liquid Soap* and *The Gold Bar* lavishly. Use *Defend Deodorant* after bathing and frequently during warm weather. Women can use *Nature's Cleanse* douche weekly if needed. Pass the "odor test" from someone in your family before you use perfumes and colognes. When serious health concerns are causing the body odor, consult your physician. Take *ProVex* or *ProVex-Plus* daily.

BOILS

Raised, red, hard, hot, and extremely painful pus-filled skin abscesses are caused by *Staphlococcus* organisms. They can appear anywhere on the body. Ears, nose, fingers, and scalp are the most painful sites due to thin skin and constant pressure. The *Staphylococcus* organism may be contracted from farm animals and it can remain dormant in the body for years before erupting, usually when the person is run down, tired, and over stressed.

Suggested Treatment: (NOTE: *Staphylococcus* is very infectious and many strains are becoming resistant to prescription antibiotics.) Apply *T36-C5* every hour to a developing boil. Some boils can be stopped at this stage. Leave exposed to the air if possible. When a focal head begins to appear, usually after a couple of days, use a sterilized needle to lance the boil and allow drainage. The release of pressure usually provides immediate relief of pain. Continue applying *T36-C5* as long as drainage lasts. If possible, soaking the site in a solution of 1 oz *Sol-U-Mel* and 2 Tbs. Epsom salts in a quart of hot water can speed drainage. Then apply *Triple Antibiotic Ointment* to a soft gauze bandage and cover. Drink 2 to 6 cups of *G'Day Melaleuca Tea* each day. Take *The Vitality Pak* with every meal. If redness and swelling does not disappear after 7 days, see your natural physician. Take *ProVex* or *ProVex-Plus* daily.

BRONCHITIS

Irritated bronchial membranes in the lung can swell and restrict air flow resulting in a condition known as bronchitis. Chronic cases can lead to asthma. Possible irritants include: low grade bacterial, yeast, or viral infections; allergies; household cleaning chemicals; and irritation from cigarette smoke. See the sections on Asthma, Chest Congestion and Coughing in this book.

Suggested Treatment: Treat the cause. Protect your air quality by converting your home to Melaleuca home care and personal care products! Take *The Vitality Pak, Cell-Wise, ProVex* or *ProVex-Plus* daily. Drink 2 to 6 cups of *G'Day Melaleuca Tea* each day. Breathe the enriched steam from a vaporizer or a bowl of steaming water each morning and night before bed. To do this, add 5 drops of *T36-C5* directly to the water. Form a tent over your head and the vaporizer or bowl, breathing the aromatic vapors through your nose and mouth gently into your lungs. Keep your eyes closed. Add 1 or 2 drops of *T36-C5* every 5 minutes for 15 to 20 minutes. For acute attacks, put 1 or 2 drops of *T36-C5* on a cotton tipped applicator and swab the inside of each nostril. (NOTE: Do not use *Sol-U-Mel* for this vaporizer treatment as it can cause irritation to the lungs.)

BRUISES

Ruptured blood vessels near the surface of the skin or in muscles can occur from injury, infection, or blood disorders. Discoloration is at first red, then black and blue, and finally green as healing takes place.

Suggested Treatment: The immediate application of ice to a traumatized area helps reduce bruising. *Pain-A-Trate* has a deep penetrating effect and reduces swelling, increases circulation, and speeds healing. Apply as often as needed until pain, discoloration, and swelling disappear. If the bruise injury is near the eye, use caution to not get the oil in or too near the eye. To prevent easy bruising and speed healing, take *ProVex*, *ProVex-Plus*, or *ProVexCV* daily. These improve the strength and elasticity of blood vessels.

BUNIONS

Bunions are caused by the swelling of the second synovial joint bursa producing enlargement and displacement of the big toe which eventually laps over the second toe. They are sometimes caused by misalignment in the spine, causing improper biomechanics in the foot. Some cases have been linked to improperly fitted shoes during childhood development. Also, see the section on Bursitis in this book.

Suggested Treatment: Apply *T36-C5* or *Pain-A-Trate* generously to the affected joint as often as discomfort exists. Soak in a solution of 1 oz *Sol-U-Mel* and 2 Tbs. of Epsom salts per quart of hot water each night. Wear only well fitting shoes, and see your local chiropractor for a walking gait analysis.

BURNS

No burn is simple to treat! This is true for a first-degree burn which is red and swollen, a second-degree burn which produces a blister, or a third-degree burn which penetrates into muscle and deep tissue and occasionally chars the flesh. Infections, scars, and even shock can result if burns are improperly treated. Too much suntanning damages skin cells. Ozone depletion in our atmosphere is increasing the amount of harmful ultraviolet rays from sunlight we are exposed to. There is an increase in melanoma skin cancer in those who are exposed to excessive ultraviolet radiation. Always protect your skin from sun exposure by using *Sun-Shades Waterproof Sunblock SPF 15* if you have dark skin, or *SPF 30* if you have a fair complexion.

Suggested Treatment: Immediately flush a fresh burn with cold water or apply ice and continue until the area is cold. Pat dry and apply *T36-C5*. Then cover with a thin coat of *Moistursil Problem Skin Lotion*. Take *ProVex* or *ProVex-Plus* daily to speed recovery and reduce scarring. Most first-degree burns will subside very soon. Repeat the *T36-C5* and *Moistursil Problem Skin Lotion* application every hour until pain is gone. For second-degree burns apply *T36-C5* and *Pain-A-Trate* immediately to prevent blistering. Repeat application of *T36-C5* and *Pain-A-Trate* each hour until pain and swelling are gone. If the burn does not show signs of healing, seek medical care. Third-degree burns require professional care immediately, since deep blood vessels, nerves, and lymphatic vessels in the skin are damaged. After cold application, apply *T36-C5* and *Moistursil Problem Skin Lotion* or *Triple Antibiotic Ointment*. Cover with a sterile covering. Contact your doctor immediately.

BURSITIS

Small fluid-filled shock absorbing sacs are present in some joints such as the elbow, knee, shoulder, hip, ankle, or big toe. Inflammation of these sacs, called bursa, causes swelling and painful movement of the joint. Trauma, infections, allergies, or toxic accumulation are the usual causes. Gradual development from repetitive motion occupations can lead to chronic bursitis. Reducing coffee drinking curiously reduces bursitis of the shoulder. Acute bursitis can result from prescription drug reactions or sudden injury to the area. See the sections on Bunions and Gout in this book.

Suggested Treatment: Take *ProVex* or *ProVex-Plus* to help reduce inflammation. Apply *Pain-A-Trate* generously to the affected area every 2 to 4 hours. Moist heat and limiting joint motion may be helpful during the healing phase. Do not exercise the joint until pain and swelling are reduced. Seek medical advice if the pain does not subside in a few days.

CALLUSES

Thickening of normal skin caused by friction, usually on the hands or feet, is seen in people whose work causes repeated pressure on a particular area. Brick layers, musicians, runners, and surfers develop typical calluses. See the sections on Corns and Warts in this book.

Suggested Treatment: Eliminate undue pressure to the affected site. Wear softer and better-fitting shoes. A moleskin or foam rubber protective bandage or arch inserts often help. *Mela-Gel* and *Moistursil Problem Skin Lotion* applied regularly helps to prevent friction at the active site. *Sole to Soul Revitalizing Foot Scrub* and *Revitalizing Foot Lotion* can also be used to cleanse and stimulate improved circulation.

CANCER PREVENTION

The second most common life threatening condition in North America is cancer. Almost one of every two citizens will develop cancer. Most will die from it in spite of the best care available. Prevention is still the wisest strategy. While no clear cause for all cancers is known, there appears to be a combination of circumstances that greatly increase the risk of cancer.

Cancer Risk = Hereditary Tendency + Carcinogen Exposure
Immune Weakness + Time

By the same token, the formula for cancer prevention is practical and sensible, which excludes it from scientific investigation and ridicule. Each one of us is responsible for our own health. Applying these simple facts to our life can give us the advantage we need. Here is the formula that many scientists agree is reasonable for preventing this dreaded disease as well as most chronic degenerative illnesses.

Cancer Prevention = Optimum Diet + Exercise & Rest
Positive Attitude + Lifetime Practice

Suggested Treatment: Whether or not you have had cancer, the recommendations included here can give you a greater measure of future cancer prevention. Many cancer researchers now believe that a combination of approaches to prevent cancer will prove to be the best treatment. Study your family tree for patterns of specific cancer types. Breast, colorectal, skin, prostate, uterus, and lung cancers seem to be more hereditary linked. Tobacco (cigarettes, pipe, smokeless tobacco), fatty diet (animal or cooked vegetable oils), toxic chemical exposure (household cleaners and personal care products, food additives, pesticides, herbicides, etc.), electromagnetic radiation (x-rays, TV, ultraviolet, etc.), and putrefying food in our digestive tract are the greatest known risks.

Get annual wellness checkups from a preventive physician. New blood tests (PSA for prostate, etc.) are being developed to detect antigens (immune sensitive chemicals) given off by early forms of cancer. Follow the doctor's recommendations.

Remove all sources of chemical exposure from your environment (especially household chemicals), and reduce your exposure to electromagnetic radiation as much as possible. Eat as if your life depended on it, because it does! Take *The Vitality Pak*, *Cell-Wise*, and *ProVex*, *ProVex-Plus*, or *ProVexCV* to ensure adequate antioxidants, B vitamins, and essential trace minerals, all of which are, to some extent, associated with cancer prevention. Men should take *ProstAvan* which contains Lycopene, which has been found to reduce the risk of prostate cancer. Drink plenty of pure water and *G'Day Melaleuca Tea* to continually detoxify. Apply *T36-C5* or *Triple Antibiotic Ointment* immediately to any suspicious skin lesion, mole, wart, skin tag, or discoloration. Continue application 2 to 4 times each day until it disappears (probably 2 to 3 weeks) or until seen by your natural physician. Laugh, sing, and play at least 30 minutes each day.

CANKER SORES

Mouth ulcers, known as canker sores, form on the gums and the inside of the cheeks. They are a localized bacterial infection characterized by a white scab appearance with a bright red border. The sores may be from pinhead size up to the size of a dime, and are very painful. They can originate from a number of causes such as damage from brushing your teeth, biting your cheek, wearing dentures, or eating hard foods. Food allergies are often linked to repeated outbreaks. See the section on Cold Sores in this book.

Suggested Treatment: Brushing with *Classic Tooth Polish* or *Fluoride Tooth Gel* and rinsing with *Breath-Away Mouthwash* reduces the bacterial count in the mouth. At the first sign of a canker sore, apply *T36-C5* to the injured site. Repeat every 4 hours.

CARBUNCLES

see Boils

CARDIOVASCULAR DISEASE

In 1912, the first case of atherosclerosis was documented in an elderly man. It was called a disease of old age, and was a novelty that took up only one paragraph of a medical textbook. By 1960, cardiovascular diseases were the number one cause of adult death in North America. The war in southeast Asia identified 19-year-old American soldiers killed in action who showed moderate to advanced plugging of the arteries in their hearts. In 1992, 485,000 Americans died from this disease. Researchers now suspect that dietary excesses and a sedentary existence may be the greatest contributors. What has happened to a people who are the envy of the world? We lack very little when compared to the rest of the world. Every president since John Kennedy has encouraged fitness proficiency in school children. Diseases such as diabetes, high LDL cholesterol, and those brought on by smoking and eating a diet low in roughage and containing over 30 percent fat, seem to be the pattern of most of those affected. Hardening of the arteries can lead to high blood pressure, shortness of breath, strokes, and cold hands and feet, as well as senility and premature aging. Oxidized cholesterol (LDL—the bad kind) and ionic calcium make up part of the "cement" which lines arteries of the liver, bowel, lungs, brain, kidneys, legs, and arms. A personal plan for prevention is needed by everyone. See the sections on Exercise and Cholesterol in this book.

Suggested Treatment: Take *ProVexCV* daily as recommended to inhibit LDL cholesterol oxidation and regulate blood platelet activity. Stop smoking and avoid smokers. Have a thorough physical examination performed to determine your risks. Follow the doctor's recommendations and chart your progress. Avoid animal fats and cooked vegetable fats. Reduce total fat to less than 20% of your total diet. Eat two green, yellow, and orange-colored vegetables each day. Begin a gradual exercise program. Eat an *Access Bar* 15 minutes before exercising to speed up the fat-burning process. Take *The Vitality Pak* and *Cell-Wise* with every meal.

CARPAL TUNNEL SYNDROME

Those who use their hands with a continual repetitive motion, such as typists, experience a thickening of the nerve sheath in their wrists causing numbness, coldness, and often pain. Any irritation from the spinal cord to the hand can accelerate the problem. Prevention is the best line of defense. B-vitamins and trace minerals are needed, and specific wrist exercises often help.

Suggested Treatment: First, eliminate the repetitive motion that caused the problem until healing is completed (often 4 to 12 weeks). Take *The Vitality Pak* with every meal. Take the saturation dose of *ProVex* or *ProVex-Plus* as directed. In addition, take *Replenex Joint Replenishing Complex* as directed. Apply *Pain-A-Trate* to the inside of the wrist and outside of the elbow every 4 hours to reduce inflammation and control pain. Avoid cold water. Hot water gives temporary relief.

CATARACTS

Damage from ultraviolet (UV) light, pollution, or steroid drugs can lead to cataracts. Free radical damage causes clouding of the lens of the eye, slowly producing fuzzy vision and a halo appearance to lights at night. Surgical treatment is more successful in the young and healthy. Nutrition and alternative therapy provide hope for many who are not able to have the surgery. Prevention is the best treatment.

Suggested Treatment: Approved UV protective lenses should be worn by everyone who is exposed to sunlight or computer monitors. Avoid animal fats, antacids, and excessive sugar. Take Melaleuca's *NutraView* as directed. Also take *The Vitality Pak* and *Cell-Wise* with each meal. *ProVex-Plus* will give additional protection for both the treatment and prevention of cataracts.

CAT SCRATCHES

Scratches from all animals, including man, promote infection. Cat scratches are among the worst, because of the high population of bacteria growing on their claws. See the section on Disinfectants in this book.

Suggested Treatment: Immediately wash the area with *Antibacterial Liquid Soap* or *The Gold Bar*. Apply a few drops of *Sol-U-Mel* to the wet wash cloth for additional disinfecting. Apply straight *T36-C5* to deep and bleeding wounds to speed drying and to slow bleeding. Apply *Triple Antibiotic Ointment* to a sterile bandage and cover. Take *ProVex* or *ProVex-Plus* daily.

CERUMEN

see Earaches

CHAPPED HANDS

see Dry Skin

CHAPPED LIPS

Wind and cold takes its toll on mucous membranes of the lips. Fevers, medications and certain health conditions that lead to dehydration often cause chapped lips.

Suggested Treatment: Cracking and pain can be prevented and restored to normal within 1 to 12 hours by applying *Sun Shades Lip Balm* every 15 to 30 minutes. *Mela-Gel* can also be used to speed recovery.

CHEST CONGESTION

Reactions to viruses, dust, allergies, mold spores, and physical activity can cause an accumulation of fluid, phlegm, or mucous in the lungs and bronchial tubes. Also read the section on Asthma in this book.

Suggested Treatment: Infections, including pneumonia, must be prevented. Irritations to the lung can rapidly develop into life-threatening conditions. Breathe the vapor from 10 drops of *T36-C5* and 2 capfuls of *Sol-U-Mel* added to a warm steam vaporizer or a bowl of steaming water. For the best results, make a tent with a towel over your head. *T36-C5* or *Pain-A-Trate* can be applied to the chest to loosen congestion. Drink adequate amounts of clear liquids including *G'Day Melaleuca Tea* and broth. Avoid mucous-forming foods such as dairy products, sugar, and wheat. While congestion exists, use *CounterAct Cold, Allergy, Sinus Medicine* as directed.

CHEST PAINS

Chest pains can be quite harmless or quite dangerous depending upon the cause. Emotional stress can cause chest tightness and localized pain. Air pollution can cause lung irritation and related chest pains. Persons who eat late in the evening, overeat, or eat in a hurry tend to have frequent indigestion and experience chest pains due to a hiatal hernia. This condition occurs when the stomach pushes up through the diaphragm due to gas in the bowel. On the other hand, when chest pain is from an occluded blood vessel, a reflex pain is usually felt extending from the chest into the left shoulder and neck area. A thorough checkup including a resting electocardiogram is recommended for active persons over 40 in an annual physical exam. Don't procrastinate! In over half of the cases of heart disease, there are no warning signs. A massive heart attack and death may be the only signs a doctor sees.

Suggested Treatment: See your natural physician if you have any chest pains! Listen to your body! Slow down when eating and eat smaller portions. Decrease your dietary fat to 20% of your total calories. Begin a progressive exercise program to maximize circulation and oxygen to the diaphragm and heart. Minimize your sugar intake, since it is directly converted into fat within your body if you do not exercise enough. Maximize your lean body mass through weight training. Make sure you eat 2 fruit servings and 5 vegetable servings every day. Take *The Vitality Pak, Cell-Wise,* and *ProVexCV* daily to insure adequate nutrient levels.

CHICKEN POX

Chicken pox is a common contagious disease of children. The incubation period is usually 14 to 21 days. The symptoms start with a skin rash. Often a fever, headache, and aching muscles are experienced. The rash changes into pimples and then blisters that enlarge and become filled with pus. The skin can become very itchy. Care should be taken to not scratch the affected areas to prevent scarring. The blisters dry up in a few days and are covered with scales. After all the blisters have scabbed, the disease is no longer contagious.

Suggested Treatment: Chicken pox is best treated by applying *T36-C5* directly on the vesicles. After the rash has fully developed, usually within 2 or 3 days, soaking in 1 oz. of *Sol-U-Mel* and 1 oz. of *Moistursil Bath Oil* in a tub of warm water for 15 minutes can help the itching. Drink one to four cups of *G'Day Melaleuca Tea* daily.

CHIGGERS

Walking through the grass in the summer in the mid-West and the South occasionally results in painful, itching eruptions on the feet, legs, and thighs. The female mite digs into the flesh and lays eggs that cause a sore. The larvae hatch and then bore under the skin causing an intense dermatitis. Read the section on Scabies in this book.

Suggested Treatment: Rub *T36-C5* on the area of the bites each morning and evening. Follow by applying *Triple Antibiotic Ointment* to prevent secondary infection. Large areas can be treated by soaking in a warm tub with 1 oz. of *Sol-U-Mel* and 1 oz. of *Moistursil Bath Oil* while scrubbing with a wash cloth and *Antibacterial Liquid Soap*. For prevention, apply *T36-C5* to the bottom of pant cuffs, or spray pants and socks with 1 oz. *Sol-U-Mel* diluted with 7 oz. of water.

CHOLESTEROL

This naturally occurring starting material for many hormones has been misunderstood mainly because of half-truths published in the news. Here is the other half of the story. There is *good* cholesterol (made from balanced nutrition during exercise and play) and *bad* cholesterol (made during stress or from over-cooked animal fats). Cholesterol is needed for life. It is our body's own antioxidant protecting us against naturally occurring free radicals. We need a certain amount of cholesterol to handle stress. We make about four times as much cholesterol in a day as we eat in our diet. Excess dietary fat (including margarine) tends to increase blood cholesterol. People who have high blood cholesterol and high stress cannot lower blood cholesterol by avoiding it in their diet. Adequate fiber and roughage in the diet carries fat and toxic substances quickly out of the body. Heat converts normal cholesterol found in animal products into oxycholesterol, which is unhealthy and toxic. The original heart disease scientists in the 1970's told us about the dangers of too much cholesterol in our blood. Today the researchers are telling us about the dangers of it being too low!

Suggested Treatment: Take *ProVexCV* daily. Take *The Vitality Pak* supplements with each meal. Begin a regular exercise program and eat an *Access Bar* 15 minutes before your workout. Put *Sustain* drink in your water (1 Tbs. per quart) while working out to maintain needed energy and electrolytes. Drink 2 to 4 cups of *G'Day Melaleuca Tea* each day.

CIGARETTE SMOKING

Imagine a 747 jumbo jet filled with passengers crashing every hour of every day within the United States borders. How long would this tragedy be allowed to continue? Of all the plagues of man, cigarette smoking has probably caused more deaths and resulted in more disease than all other non-infectious causes combined. Over 50 toxic or banned substances have been identified resulting from smoking; these include carbon monoxide, carbon dioxide, dioxane, arsenic oxide, biphenyls, and cadmium salts, just to name a few. Nicotine, after the Latin name of the plant meaning nightshade, is a powerful insect repellent, aphid killer on roses, and deadly poison which is never eaten by animals in the wild. Smoking one cigarette reduces the infection-fighting ability of the immune system by 50 percent for 2 hours. It has been advised against by the March Of Dimes since 1974 for causing birth defects. Second-hand smoke has been linked to a 15% lower IQ among children of households where at least one parent is a smoker. Nicotine is an addictive alkaloid drug related to codeine, morphine, and cocaine. Recently, cigarette companies have been accused of actually adding nicotine to their higher priced brands to induce greater addiction and desire for their product. Many congressmen list financial holdings in the lucrative tobacco industry, which may account for the 30-year struggle to gain governmental bans of this deadly waste of human health.

Suggested Treatment: There is no greater single health measure you can take than to quit smoking and forbid the practice in your home or around your loved ones. Like any drug addiction, it must be faced with courage and compassion. If you have the personal strength to stop smoking—do it right now! If you need help, seek a natural physician who is trained in chemical addiction treatment with diet, herbs, acupuncture and hypnosis. Begin a lifestyle of wellness rather than self-destruction. Take *ProVex, ProVex-Plus,* or *ProVexCV* daily. Take *The Vitality Pak* and *Cell-Wise* every meal. Drink 2 to 4 cups of *G'Day Melaleuca Tea* each day.

COLD SORES

Very painful clear, fluid-filled eruptions on the border of the mouth form hard, oozing scabs resulting from an infection of either the herpes simplex or herpes facialis virus. Once thought to be more common in infants and children, adults are becoming more susceptible. The infection makes chewing difficult and may impede the appetite. Mild damage associated with exposure to the sun, stress, abrasions from a toothbrush, bad allergies to certain foods, the onset of menstruation, or any disease that produces a fever or increases metabolic rate may produce a lesion. As a rule, the symptoms generally go away after 7 to 10 days. Dehydration and secondary infections give reason for concern.

Suggested Treatment: Since the virus feeds on an excessive intake of the amino acid *arginine*, diets avoiding citrus fruit and nuts should be followed. Supplementation with the amino acid L-Lysine, found in most health food stores, is advised to stop the early spread of the infection. Dab *T36-C5* on the lesions immediately upon detection. Repeat every hour until the lesion either disappears or comes to a head. If it comes to a head, continue to apply *T36-C5* once every 2 hours followed by *Mela-Gel* or *Moistursil Problem Skin Lotion*. For persistent or large surface sores, use *Triple Antibiotic Ointment* every 4 hours. See also the section on "Canker Sores."

COLIC

Chronic severe abdominal pain can be caused from a number of conditions that may be non-life-threatening. See the section on Appendicitis in this book. Newborns may experience colic when the digestive system has not developed enough to handle food properly. Gas or constipation is the usual cause of the abdominal pain. Heavy metal poisoning (lead, copper, zinc, cadmium, etc.), food or environmental allergies, ovarian cysts, gallstones, kidney stones, intestinal parasites, pesticide residue from produce, food poisoning, chlorine poisoning, and chronic constipation can all cause colic.

Suggested Treatment: Get a thorough examination from your natural physician to identify the cause, if possible. Chiropractic adjustments can be quite effective in giving relief. *Pro-Vex* can also give relief. A hot moist pack with *Pain-A-Trate* on the affected area can be beneficial. Soak fruits and vegetables in 2 quarts of cold water and 1/2 tsp. of *Sol-U-Mel* for 10 minutes, then rinse in pure water. Detoxify by using only steamed and juiced vegetables at least one meal each day. Drink 1 to 2 quarts of water, plus 2 to 4 cups of *G'Day Melaleuca Tea* per day. Take the *This is Fiber?!* bars as a snack. Exercise regularly.

For the infant suffering from colic, there are several treatments to consider. The food source is the first possible problem. Mother's milk is best for an infant, at least for the first year. If colic is present, the mother may need to be careful not to eat any rich, spicy, or gas-forming foods. Also, if she is experiencing stress, her milk may be affected, so stay calm and get plenty of rest. Do not introduce any other foods for the baby until advised by a natural physician. If the baby is drinking formula, he may be having an allergic food reaction. A change in formula may be needed. Gas is a common cause of colic. Gently but firmly patting the baby on his back or bottom should help eliminate the gas. Giving the baby a pacifier may help reduce tension and colic. If constipation is a serious concern, a physician will suggest some possible solutions for the baby.

To correct colic in infants, give several teaspoons of warm *G'Day Melaleuca Tea* during the day and before bed. Many infants have also found relief when given *ProVex* once daily. Simply open a capsule and dissolve the *ProVex* in distilled water, juice, or expressed breast milk. Chiropractic adjustments are also effective for correction of colic in infants.

COMMON COLD

Cold viruses attack the moist, cooler regions of the nose, throat, sinuses, vocal cords, and larynx when our systems are run down. The virus has developed a way of avoiding destruction by the immune system and is present in a dormant state. Apparently, when we contact a cold from someone else (sneeze, handshake, kiss), the two viruses exchange fragments of genetic information to form a slightly new strain. It is new enough to enter living cells undetected where it begins to multiply until cell damage has taken place and the immune system drives the virus into seclusion until the next opportune time arises. Mucous membranes become swollen, red and irritated as the virus spreads from one cell to the next. Untreated colds can progress into more threatening conditions.

Suggested Treatment: The common cold usually gives a warning that it is about to develop. From the earliest signs of tiredness, sneezing, and hoarseness you are given a few hours to launch an attack. Immediately take *Activate Immune Complex* as directed, and take a hot bath. Take

CounterAct Cold, Allergy, Sinus Medicine as directed. Also, breathe the steamy vapor of five drops of *T36-C5* and water in a steam inhaler for fifteen minutes (air temperatures above 104 degrees kill the virus). Apply one drop of *T36-C5* to each nostril of your nose every four hours. Sip vegetable broth and/or mom's chicken soup every couple of hours. Avoid any temptation to eat heavy foods as your digestive tract, including smell and taste, are on vacation for awhile. If coughing is present, use *CounterAct Cough Relief Medicine* as directed. Try a hot *Sustain* drink to fight any fever you may produce. To reduce painful muscles, take *Mela-Cal* four times a day and bathe with *Moistursil Bath Oil* frequently. "Drown the cold" with *G'Day Melaleuca Tea* — one cup per hour. Get all the rest you can.

COMPRESSION FRACTURES

Automobile accidents, athletic injuries, falls, chronic muscle spasms, and decreased bone calcium (see Osteoporosis) can cause the vertebrae of the spine to squeeze together with sufficient force to break the bone. After the age of 25, very little blood circulation is available to properly heal the injury.

Suggested Treatment: See your natural physician for professional care. Diagnosis of compression fractures requires an x-ray. Take *Mela-Cal* 3 to 6 times per day to minimize pain from muscle spasms. Apply *Pain-A-Trate* to the affected muscles and gently, but firmly, massage above and below the affected area. Take *ProVex* or *ProVex-Plus* daily for quicker healing.

CONJUNCTIVITIS

An irritation of the pink skin flap of the eyelid can be caused by a bacterial infection (often contagious), allergy (itching and burning), or chemical contact (red and painful). Children often get contagious *"pink eye"* from playmates. Consult your natural physician.

Suggested Treatment: Great relief can come simply from rinsing the eye in warm distilled water several times a day. Often this one treatment will allow the eyelid to heal. Some have had good success treating mild conjunctivitis in the early stage by putting 5 drops of *T36-C5* in a warm steam vaporizer and slowly blinking the eyes carefully in the direct path of the vapor. Repeat every 5 minutes for three consecutive doses before bed. Repeat morning and night for 3 days. If the irritation persists, see your natural physician. Take *ProVex* or *ProVex-Plus* daily. Note: Do not put any *Melaleuca* products directly on the eye. Use only products that are certified ophthamologic grade.

CONSTIPATION

It is healthy and normal to have a bowel movement within one to two hours after eating. Wastes, including undigested fiber, pass out of the healthy body within 12 hours after eating the meal. Poor diet, lack of exercise, not drinking enough water, stress, and many drugs can cause constipation. We are a constipated society. Colorectal diseases are at an epidemic level. See the section on Hemorrhoids in this book.

Suggested Treatment: The following four things help most sufferers of constipation: eat enough fiber, drink enough liquids, get enough exercise to maintain bowel mobility, and don't worry so much. Specifically, get 20 to 30 grams of fiber each day. (Note: 1 medium apple + 1/2 cup of old fashioned oatmeal + 1/4 cup raisins + 2 carrots + 1 cup of broccoli + 1/2 cup of cooked beans = 10 grams of fiber). Take the *This is Fiber?!* bars to maximize fiber. Drink 1 to 3 quarts of water including *G'Day Melaleuca Tea* each day. Take *ProVex* or *ProVex-Plus* daily. Run, walk, jog, bike or swim, etc. for 30 minutes each day. Replace thoughts of fear or worry with happy, optimistic thoughts. This releases hormones in the bowel which aid digestive juices and propel food along the bowel and out of the body.

CORAL CUTS

Coral cuts are often jagged and irregular, and they harbor bacteria. This necessitates thorough cleansing and disinfecting. See the section on Disinfectants in this book.

Suggested Treatment: Thoroughly cleanse with pure water and *Antibacterial Liquid Soap* enriched with *Sol-U-Mel*. Remove particles of sand and coral. Apply *T36-C5* or *T40-C3* for maximum disinfecting. Suturing wounds that cut through the skin and into muscle speeds healing and reduces secondary infection. Apply *Triple Antibiotic Ointment* over the stitches, if applicable, and cover with a gauze bandage. Daily inspect the wound for redness or swelling, which gives indication of the spread of infection. When sutures are not needed, soak affected areas in a solution of 1oz. *Sol-U-Mel*, plus 1 oz. *Moistursil Bath Oil*, plus 1/4 cup Epsom salt in 1 quart of hot water. Rinse open wounds daily with 1 oz. of *Sol-U-Mel* in 1 pint of water. Change the dressing daily and reapply *Triple Antibiotic Ointment* or *Mela-Gel*.

CORNS

Corns are raised areas of hyperkeratosis or thick callused skin which are caused by friction or pressure often over a bony extension of the foot, such as the ball of the foot or the toe joints. Corns are first noticed as pea size or slightly larger and occur on the side and bottom of the feet. Hard corns occur over the toes and soft corns occur between the toes. Corns may ache spontaneously or become very tender upon pressure. Proper fitting shoes will help prevent corns. See the section on Calluses in this book.

Suggested Treatment: Soak feet in a solution of 1 oz. *Sol-U-Mel* and 1 oz. *Moistursil Bath Oil* in 1 quart of hot water for 15 minutes. Proceed twice daily until the corn softens enough to remove the core with tweezers. Apply *Triple Antibiotic Ointment* or *Mela-Gel* and cover with a small bandage. *Sole to Soul Revitalizing Foot Scrub* and *Revitalizing Foot Lotion* can also be used to cleanse and stimulate improved circulation. Wear only shoes that fit properly.

CORYZA

see Common Cold

COUGHING

Our bodies produce phlegm and mucous in the throat and lungs when exposed to severe temperature changes, chemical irritation, or allergens. We instinctively cough to remove this phlegm and foreign substances. Smoking is the most common cause of chronic coughs. See the section on Smoking in this book. Severe coughing can cause bleeding of the throat or inner ear infections.

Suggested Treatment: Treat the cause—eliminate your exposure to the irritating substances. In mild cases, breathe the vapor of 5 drops of *T36-C5* in a bowl of steaming water for 15 minutes while holding your head over the bowl. Make a tent over your head and the bowl with a bath towel. Repeat morning and evening. Drink the *G'Day Melaleuca Tea* throughout the day. Use *CounterAct Cough Relief Medicine* as directed. If congestion exists, use *CounterAct Allergy/Sinus* as directed.

CRACKED SKIN

see Dry Skin

CRAMPS

Sudden decreases in tissue oxygen, decreases in muscle or nerve calcium levels, or hormonal changes before menstrual flow can trigger muscle cramps. Side aches during or after strenuous exercise are due to diaphragm spasms caused from low oxygen and low calcium levels in that muscle.

Suggested Treatment: After eating a meal, wait 45 minutes before exercising. Properly stretch and warm muscles before exercise. *Mela-Cal* taken 4 times per day and at bedtime can prevent sub-optimum levels of calcium in the blood and prevent cramps. Eat an *Access Bar* 15 minutes before exercise. Drink *Sustain* drink during and immediately after exercise. A warm bath and a good massage can help reduce pain greatly. Massage *Pain-A-Trate* into muscles which cramp easily. The therapeutic dose of *ProVex* (1 capsule for every 25 pounds of body weight per day) can also give good relief, as can *CounterAct Extra-Strength Acetaminophen* or *Ibuprofen*.

CUTICLES

The rolled skin at the edge of the finger and toe nails can give evidence of your general health. Dry cuticles which split and become infected are often due to exposure to harsh soaps or solvents such as gasoline or paint thinner. See the section on Dry Skin in this book.

Suggested Treatment: After washing hands with *Antibacterial Liquid Soap* or *The Gold Bar*, apply *Hand Creme* to the hands and work into the cuticles to prevent dryness. Apply *Triple Antibiotic Ointment* or *Mela-Gel* to infected cuticles. If condition persists, see your natural physician.

CUTS

If the object that caused the injury was dirty or exposed to disease-causing organisms, extra care must be taken in thorough cleaning. Cuts should be treated soon after injury.

Suggested Treatment: Clean the affected area with a wash cloth, warm water, and *Antibacterial Liquid Soap* and/or *Sol-U-Mel*. Apply *T36-C5* and keep clean with a bandage. Check the healing progress daily. Re-clean and apply new bandages as often as needed. Deep or wide cuts may require a visit to your natural physician for suturing.

DANDRUFF

This dry flaking of the scalp is one of the most common conditions affecting the adult population. White, scaly skin sloughs off of the head in a "*snow storm*" fashion to disgrace the victim. The use of poor quality soaps and shampoos can irritate the sebaceous (oil) glands and produce a dry scalp that flakes off when combing or brushing. The condition upsets the normal healthy skin bacteria and adds the typical itch to the unsightly condition. Because of our chemical and perfumed countenance, dandruff proliferates.

Suggested Treatment: Avoid harsh soaps, shampoos, and hair care products. Shampoo with *Natural Shampoo* or *Melaleuca Essentials Shampoo*.

DEAFNESS

Gradual loss of hearing in adults can be due to the incurable condition of nerve loss caused from viruses, infections, high fevers, prescription drugs, and trauma. One estimate is that 20 percent of the adult population is hearing-impaired. Partial hearing loss can often be helped with hearing aids. Some adults go through the best years of their lives never knowing what they are missing.

Generally over one half of adults have accumulated wax in one or both ears, which impedes hearing to some extent. Earwax cleaning is an important preventive practice for small children as well as adults. Some recurring middle ear infections in children permanently disappear when the ears are kept clean. Some people need their ears cleaned as often as once or twice a year.

Suggested Treatment: To remove excess earwax that may be interfering with hearing, follow the treatment directions in the section on Earwax in this book. Get a hearing test from a qualified audiologist.

DECAYED TEETH

Dentists have done an admirable job in helping prevent tooth decay. Brushing, flossing, and swishing after eating has become a way of life for most of us. Nonetheless, some decay still takes place. Dentists and scientists argue that the use of fluoride, while definitely reducing tooth decay in some, may pose a greater risk in the long run to the general health of the body.

Refined foods (mainly sugar in its many forms) promote rapid yeast, bacterial, and other microorganism growth in the many cracks and crevices in and around the teeth. These microbes secrete acids which erode the calcium-rich enamel of the teeth. Proper brushing and flossing habits are essential to reduce the microbial population.

Suggested Treatment: Gently brush the teeth and tongue after every meal with *Classic Tooth Polish*. Swish mouth with *Breath-Away Mouthwash* to reduce mouth microbes as well as to control jungle breath. Floss frequently with *Exceed* and chew *Insta-Fresh* gum frequently. Take *ProVex* or *ProVex-Plus* to help prevent plaque buildup. Have regular checkups with your dentist to maintain healthy teeth.

DECIDUOUS TEETH

see Baby Teeth

DEPRESSION (MILD)

One of the most common conditions experienced by adults and young people is occasional depression—an attitude that "I don't feel like doing what I normally would like to do." It is normal for someone to feel blue or have an attitude of melancholy from time to time due to undesirable situations. It is another thing to see a black cloud cast over the future. Some people actually develop a sort of regular "gloom and doom" attitude if depression is allowed to persist. Nutritional deficiencies or fast foods often provoke such feelings. Exposure to household chemicals and food additives may also contribute. If a cause for the depressed mood can be identified, then the cause should be treated. Menopause can also increase the need for estrogen stabilization to control mild depression.

Suggested Treatment: Having a positive support group during times of depression is of great benefit. Take *Luminex* along with *The Vitality Pak*, *ProVex-Plus* or *ProVexCV*, and *Cell-Wise*. *EstrAval* can be taken as directed to reduce mild depression during the change of life. Harmful household chemicals should be eliminated and replaced with biologically safe ones. Drinking 1 to 2 cups of *G'Day Melaleuca Tea* daily and eating and exercising regularly each day can be very helpful.

DERMATITIS

Inflammation of the skin with redness, oozing, crusting, scaling, and sometimes vesicles can be sudden and short-lived or chronic in nature. More than 50 percent of all skin conditions I see in my practice can be classified as dermatitis. Chronic dermatitis is commonly known as eczema.

Healthy skin is able to withstand exposure to many natural substances and some synthetic chemicals without harmful effects (it is designed to be our first line of defense against the outside world.) Substances which irritate the skin include plants such as poison ivy, some trees, some fruits and vegetables, therapeutic drugs such as cortisone and antibiotic creams, cosmetics and hair dyes, fabrics such as wool and synthetics, as well as toxic household cleaners and chemicals. In addition to these external sources, there are internal conditions such as allergies and sensitivities to foods and prescription and over-the-counter drugs that often cause dermatitis.

Suggested Treatment: Reduce the amount of toxins in the air in your home by converting your home to Melaleuca cleaning and personal care products. Many cases of dermatitis are greatly reduced by switching to the *EcoSense Laundry System* and laundering all clothing, linens, and towels. Try to identify the cause of the dermatitis before aggressively treating the symptoms. As soon as possible after the symptoms begin, wash the area with *Antibacterial Liquid Soap* or *The Gold Bar*. Additional soaking in a warm tub with 1 oz. of *Sol-U-Mel* and 1 oz. of *Moistursil Bath Oil* once daily is advised. Use *Moistursil Problem Skin Lotion* twice daily. *Triple Antibiotic Ointment* is also effective.

DIABETES

Juvenile-onset diabetes appears to be due to a defective gene that causes self-destruction of insulin-producing cells in the pancreas. Insulin must then be taken regularly to support life. Adult-onset diabetes, on the other hand, appears to be due to suppression or inhibition of normal pancreas production. Being over 55 years of age and overweight, lacking exercise, and consuming large amounts of refined sugar and dietary fat (more than 20% of daily calories) is the typical picture. Usually, insulin is unnecessary but a pancreatic stimulant drug is often prescribed.

Suggested Treatment: Drink 2 to 4 cups of *G'Day Melaleuca Tea* each day, and take *The Vitality Pak* and *Cell-Wise* with each meal. Take *ProVex-Plus* at the therapeutic dose level (one capsule per 25 pounds of body weight daily) or *ProVexCV* daily as directed. This increases circulation and reduces the incidence of many diabetic symptoms. These supplements are also very important to protect the eyesight of diabetics. Blood sugar levels can be somewhat regulated using the *Access Bars* and/or *Sustain*. Make exercise and a low-fat, low-sugar diet a way of life. For best mouth health, use *Classic Tooth Polish, Exceed* floss, and *Breath-Away* at least twice daily. For quickest healing of wounds, use *Mela-Gel* and *T36-C5*.

DIAPER RASH

Common diaper rash is caused by friction and irritation in the presence of moisture, which triggers yeast to grow. This occurs naturally when wet diapers are not changed promptly. Hospital nurseries often harbor resistant strains of these organisms. You may bring them home with your new bundle of joy. Elderly or incontinent adults must also beware of this problem.

Suggested Treatment: Properly launder all baby clothing as well as diapers in hot water enriched with 1 oz. of *Sol-U-Mel* per load. *Sol-U-Mel* should not be used in bath water as the green soap in it may irritate sensitive skin (newborn babies lack active sweat glands.) *Antibacterial Liquid Soap* or *The Gold Bar* should be used to bathe your baby. After towel drying your baby, allow skin to air dry (in direct sunlight if possible) for a few minutes. Apply *Moistursil Problem Skin Lotion*, *Body Satin Lotion* or *Hand Creme* to form a natural moisture barrier on the skin before diapering.

DIARRHEA

A sudden increase in stool volume, fluidity, or frequency of fecal excretion is seen with microbial infections, flu viruses, stress, food poisoning, laxatives, certain genetic and malabsorption problems, and electrolyte loss from vomiting or drugs. The greatest concern is depletion of body fluid resulting in vascular collapse (the heart has nothing to pump). Children under the age of 4 can dehydrate quickly and die from uncontrolled diarrhea.

Suggested Treatment: Determine the cause, if possible. If there is abdominal pain, fever, or if the diarrhea does not resolve rapidly, seek emergency help without delay. Otherwise, begin drinking *G'Day Melaleuca Tea*, 4 to 16 oz. every hour along with *Sustain* drink for energy and nutrient replacement.

DISINFECTANTS

Disinfectants work by selectively reducing the population of disease-causing germs to make room for the friendly germs without harming humans or household plants and animals. Sanitation engineers have taught us that in order to control the spread of disease, we must control the number and transportability of disease causing germs. Several products are effective and especially stand out for their use in making safe play-toys, furniture, clothing, and bodies. See the Appendix in the back of this book for a comparison of the disinfectant properties of *T36-C5* compared to other agents.

Suggested Treatment: Sponge-bathe a sick person with *Antibacterial Liquid Soap* or *The Gold Bar* on a wash cloth to reduce surface germs often transported through perspiration. Rinse well. Disinfect the air by running a warm steam vaporizer with 10 drops *T36-C5* and 2 capfuls of *Sol-U-Mel* in the sickroom. For preventing the spread of germs through the skin, use *Clear Defense* throughout the day to sanitize and kill germs on hands without the need for soap and water. A general disinfectant solution for cleaning a sickroom is a solution of 1 oz. *MelaPower* laundry detergent plus 1 oz. *Sol-U-Mel* in 1 gallon of warm water. Sponge, mop, or wipe floors, walls, doorknobs, lamps, and bed frames.

DIVERTICULOSIS

Chronic constipation, insufficient fluid intake, inadequate dietary roughage, and some medications can cause pressure in the lower bowel sufficient to cause bulges or sacs in the muscular wall. These bulging pockets, or diverticuli, can become impacted with fecal material and extend to over one inch in length. If improperly cared for, they can develop irritation, pain, and serious infections—a condition known as diverticulosis.

Suggested Treatment: Until about 20 years ago, a low roughage diet was recommended for treating diverticulosis. Puddings, white bread, Jell-O and soft vegetables proved, however, to do little to stop the surgeon's knife. Oat bran, wheat bran, and psyllium, along with adequate exercise and liquids are the treatment of choice for diverticulosis. Adequate roughage found in *This is Fiber?!* and *G'Day Melaleuca Tea*, 2 to 4 cups per day, is a good way to increase bowel elimination and reduce pressure. *The Vitality Pak*, *Cell-Wise*, and *ProVex* are needed for healing and improved health.

DIZZINESS

Most of us have experienced motion sickness when we whirl around, ride a merry-go-round, or go out on the ocean in a small boat. The feeling that objects are moving around us tricks our equilibrium mechanism in the inner ear and can even be due to an optical illusion (Omni Vision). Several health conditions can make us susceptible to this feeling such as middle ear infections, tumors, toxicity from drugs or alcohol, brain injuries, and concussions. One of the most common causes of unexplained dizziness is from low blood sugar in reactive hypoglycemia or after exercise. Diabetics can get it from insulin reactions.

Suggested Treatment: See your natural health doctor if unexplained dizziness is occurring. For blood sugar control, eat small meals often throughout the day instead of large meals eaten less often. Avoid sugary foods, since this causes sudden drops in blood glucose from the rebounding insulin release. Take *The Vitality Pak* and *ProVex* supplements daily. Eat an *Access Bar* 15 minutes before exercise so your body can burn fats instead of running out of fuel. If you get dizzy easily during or after exercise, drink *Sustain* drink in your water while working out.

DRUG POISONING

Three out of every ten hospital admissions are due to either prescription or over-the-counter drug reactions. Sixteen hundred people die each year from aspirin poisoning alone. Be certain that your drug-oriented doctor communicates all possible side effects from any needed medications. Eli Lily, pharmacist and founder of Lily Pharmaceuticals is quoted as saying, *"A drug without side effects—is no drug at all."* Dermatitis, nausea, accelerated heart rate, excessive sweating, stomach pains, and diarrhea are some of the milder reactions. Tumors, kidney failure, diabetes, ulcers, and sudden death are the more common severe reactions. One pharmacist friend of mine says that only one third of prescriptions are taken in the proper dosage or for the duration that they are prescribed. Other authorities state that the overuse of prescription antibiotics has resulted in superresistant strains of bacteria which defy all known treatment and killed over 13,000 hospitalized patients in 1992 alone.

Some drugs react with others to produce baffling symptoms. When several doctors are treating the same patient for different conditions, the risk of drug interactions increases. The most recent Physicians Desk Reference lists over 2300 reactions from drugs—many from misuse. Be informed and realize that the majority of drugs are for *"treating symptoms"* only and do not offer a cure! If your doctor says you will need to take the drug for the rest of your life, he or she is often referring to this philosophy. Only the body can cure! Prevention and common sense can reduce the need for many drugs and their potential side effects on us and on our environment.

Suggested Treatment: Always ask your medical doctor or pharmacist to list the possible side effects of the prescription drugs you are asked to take. Drink *G'Day Melaleuca Herbal Tea* every hour to speed detoxification. Take *The Vitality Pak*, along with *ProVex* or *ProVex-Plus* daily to help detoxification.

DRY SKIN

Some people have dry skin due to hormonal or nutrient deficiencies, prescription medications, or a deficiency of essential fatty acids in their diet. Hands that work in caustic or cold environments or those that are washed frequently (food handlers or healthcare workers) will develop excessively dry, cracked skin. Women who are going through the change of life are very prone to dry skin and chapped hands. The decreased production of natural oils reduces moisture in skin.

Suggested Treatment: Wash in *Antibacterial Liquid Soap*, then apply *Moistursil Problem Skin Lotion* liberally. Apply *Triple Antibiotic Ointment* or *Mela-Gel* to cracked or infected areas. *Hand Creme* can be used on hands after washing to help restore moisture. When hand chapping has begun, apply *Moistursil Problem Skin Lotion* every 4 hours until normal skin moisture is restored. Skin dryness that has invaded deeper tissues or caused swelling will require treatment with *Triple Antibiotic Ointment* every 4 hours. This will help to control infection until healing is accomplished. *Pain-A-Trate* has been used by some patients with poor circulation. Take *The Vitality Pak* with every meal and take *ProVex* or *ProVex-Plus* each day to help improve skin suppleness and elasticity.

DUODENAL ULCERS

see Gastric Ulcers

DYSENTERY

see Diarrhea

EAR INFECTIONS

Repeated ear infections with fever and pain (see Earaches) requiring cycles of antibiotics are a sign of continual blockage of the ear canal. Infections of the outer ear (pinna) can travel into the ear canal where severe pain is produced. Permanent hearing loss or meningitis can result if treatment is delayed. If antibiotics are unsuccessful, tiny Teflon tubes are often surgically inserted through the eardrum, which allow accumulating fluid and pus to drain outward from the ear. The tubes are occasionally expelled within a few days or weeks and constitute a major part of some pediatricians' practices. Other pediatricians refuse to use this technique because of questionable results and the rare chance that they may travel deeper into the middle ear to create new problems. Swimmers, bottle-fed infants, and recently immunized children frequently experience ear infections.

Suggested Treatment: Don't overlook allergies as a cause. Identify the cause, if possible. See your natural physician if in doubt. (NOTE: The American Lung Association cites formaldehyde as a possible major cause of chronic ear infection in children. Formaldehyde is an ingredient in many cleaning and personal care products commonly found in the home.) Never send a child with an ear infection outdoors if the air is cool.

To treat an ear infection, use a drop of *T36-C5* or *T40-C3* mixed with 12 to 15 drops of warm olive oil or other neutral oil to saturate the end of a cotton plug. Carefully insert the plug directly into the outside ear canal and leave overnight. (CAUTION: A cotton plug could become a choke hazard for very small children and babies. Instead, insert the oil mixture directly into the outside ear canal with a dropper 3-4 times daily.) Avoid using full strength *T36-C5* in ears as local irritation can result. A hot water bottle or heating pad set on low should be put over the ear. Drink 4 to 16 ounces of *G'Day Melaleuca Tea* every hour to prevent dehydration from the fever. If congestion exists, use *CounterAct Cold/Allergy/Sinus* as directed.

EARWAX

Some people produce more earwax than others. Some people also produce hard wax while others make soft earwax. There is some relationship between excessive earwax production and high blood lipids (cholesterol or triglycerides). Earwax may plug the ear canal and cause itching, pain, and temporary hearing loss.

Suggested Treatment: To clean excess or impacted wax from the ear canal, do the following. Apply one drop of *T36-C5* and one drop of *Sol-U-Mel* to a small piece of cotton which has been pulled and twisted to a point. Insert the soaked point in the ear canal overnight. The next morning, remove the cotton and fill a rubber baby syringe (purchased at any drug store) with a solution of 1 tsp. *Sol-U-Mel* in 8 ounces of water heated to body temperature. Hold the syringe toward the side of the canal just inside the ear opening, leaving a space for the water to swish back out. Squeeze a firm stream of water into the ear canal several times to melt and dislodge the wax. NOTE: Old wax may require the application of a heating pad to the ear for about 10 minutes before irrigating. If the wax is too hard or too large, consult your natural physician.

EARACHES

Unlike adults, the ear canal in infants and small children inclines upward from the inner ear toward its exit in the throat. This anatomical uphill climb makes children more susceptible to earaches and inner ear infections. You do not have to have infection to have earaches. Milk drinking after weaning, allergies, the common cold, and even teething can cause this problem. Symptomatic relief is often given with antihistamines, aspirin, and Tylenol. A cool breeze can set off ear canal muscle spasms. Many foreign substances have been removed from children's ear canals including beans, beads, blueberries, a live moth (very painful), and rocks. Using cotton tipped swabs to clean the ears can push wax and other materials to the back of the ear canal against the eardrum, causing damage. Rapid changes in air pressure (such as landing in an airplane) quickly identify the children and adults who have Eustachian tube congestion.

Suggested Treatment: Determine the cause of the pain, if possible. Cover a child's ears when out in cold or windy weather to prevent earaches. Loose cotton pushed into the outer ear canal can help protect sensitive ears. Holding the open end of Styrofoam cups firmly over the ears when landing an airplane has a dramatic effect on preventing earaches in adults as well as children. A drop of warm *T36-C5* or *T40-C3* can be mixed with 5 to 10 drops of olive oil or other neutral oil to saturate the end of a cotton plug. This inserted in the outside ear canal and left overnight will help minimize pain. Avoid using straight oil in sensitive ears as local irritation can result. Diluted warm *T36-C5* can be dripped into an ear that has a live bug inside. This will kill the bug so it can be removed painlessly. If congestion exists, use *CounterAct Cold/Sinus/Allergy* as directed.

ECZEMA

see Dermatitis

EDEMA

Hot weather, lack of exercise, kidney, liver, or heart problems as well as drug toxicity can cause swelling due to excessive sodium and water retention. Sudden weight gain of 2 to 15 pounds in a few days may be the first signal. Obesity, fatty diet, salty foods, carbonated beverages, and excessive sugar tend to increase edema. Lower legs, ankles, and feet are the most often affected. Facial puffiness usually denotes kidney disease. One way to test for edema is to press on the inside of the ankle with moderate finger pressure. If a *"pit"* is seen when pressure is released, this means there is excessive fluid trapped in the space between cells. Edema that develops only toward the end of the day most often responds to diet, exercise, and stress control.

Suggested Treatment: Exercise regularly. Drink 2 to 6 cups of *G'Day Melaleuca Herbal Tea* each day and take *The Vitality Pak, Cell-Wise,* and *ProVex* or *ProVex-Plus* with each meal. Elevate the legs for 15 minutes in the mid-afternoon and evening. Wear support hose when standing or walking for prolonged periods.

EMPHYSEMA

Mature adults who have been exposed to air pollutants or who have smoked develop this illness. The germ and pollution digesting enzymes that are released by the white blood cells cause permanent damage to the tiny air sacs in the lung. The person has trouble exhaling and develops an enlarged or over-extended chest. A simple spirometry test (lung volume) and history usually tell a story of hard work and an abused life. If the person also has allergies, further development of asthma is common. See the sections on Air Purification, Asthma, and Bronchitis in this book.

Suggested Treatment: Treatment to prevent further damage includes stopping smoking, getting moderate exercise unless the heart is also damaged, drinking 2 to 4 cups of *G'Day Melaleuca Tea* daily, and taking *The Vitality Pak*, *Cell-Wise*, and *ProVex* or *ProVex-Plus* with each meal. Steam inhalation each night with a few drops of *T36-C5* is helpful to prevent infections from bacteria, yeast and fungus. Follow the directions under the section on Bronchitis in this book. If congestion exists, use *CounterAct Cold/Sinus/Allergy* as directed. It is most important to remove toxins from the home by converting to Melaleuca personal care and home care products. Use *Sol-U-Mel* to clean all equipment.

ENLARGED PROSTATE

see Benign Prostatic Hyperplasia (BPH)

EXERCISE

Why should we exercise? Because we are designed to be physical creatures as well as emotional and spiritual ones. A better word for this activity is play! Children expend more daily calories per kilogram of their body weight than adults because of their attitude about play. The purpose of exercise is to improve the efficiency of combining oxygen with fuel to produce energy. In the clinical laboratory this is measured as the VO_2 max, (maximum volume of oxygen used per unit time). The word *aerobics* (done with oxygen) describes exercises that tend to improve or condition the body to do this more efficiently. In order to achieve the greatest benefit, an exercise must be chosen which is enjoyable, comfortable, and ideally performed at a level of exertion at which a casual conversation can be maintained. Physically exhausting activities should be avoided if better health is the goal. Having an exercise target helps to get the most from your activity. Your target heart rate is based on an equation developed by exercise scientists. You must have a watch with a second hand and be able to take your pulse in your wrist or feel it in your neck.

220 - Your Age x 0.8 = Your Target Heart Rate

Example: If you are 50 years old,

220 - 50 x 0.8 = 136 beats/minute
(about 14 beats in 6 seconds)

This is 80% of your maximum attainable heart rate (at 100%, your heart is put under too much stress). Exercise helps to reduce the resting heart rate. The most complete body exercises are swimming, jumping on a trampoline, and cross-country skiing, because they use so many muscles. The next best exercises are walking, hiking, jogging, soccer, bicycling, aerobic dancing and skating. Court sports such as tennis, racquetball, handball, basketball and volleyball are good, but do not keep the heart rate even enough to sustain the conditioning effect. Other activities usually need to be included in your weekly work out schedule if you want better overall health. Weight lifting, bowling, archery, baseball, and horseback riding are more anaerobic (done without oxygen) and are great sports, but they cannot provide the kind of activity to keep the blood and oxygen adequately supplied to all organs of the body. Always make sure that you have adequate hydration before you start to exercise (I drink 1 quart of liquid before each daily work out.)

Suggested Treatment: Take *Vitality Pak, Cell-Wise,* and *ProVex or ProVex-Plus* with each meal, or *ProVexCV* as directed. Eat an *Access Bar* 15 minutes before exercise. Drink water throughout and after exercise.

EXERCISE STRAIN

There are several levels of muscle strain. Mild strain occurs regularly with all forms of exercise. Severe muscle strains can cause tearing and bruising. See the section on Bruises in this book.

Suggested Treatment: Overused muscles, tendons (connecting muscles to bones), and ligaments (connecting bones to other bones) are helped by immediately applying ice to prevent swelling. Keep the ice on for 5 to 10 minutes each hour, until the swelling is reduced. *Pain-A-Trate* gives dramatic relief from athletic strains.

EYE INJURIES

Never put *T36-C5*, *Triple Antibiotic Ointment*, or *Mela-Gel* in the eye as they can cause pain and dryness of the eyeball. None of the medicine chest products are approved for use in the eye. Read the section on Bruises in this book.

Suggested Treatment: None of the Melaleuca products are approved for use in or near the eye. If the injury is due to caustic chemicals splashing in the eye, you should immediately wash the eye with fresh water for several minutes. Contact your eye doctor without delay. Foreign matter in the eye can scratch or even penetrate the cornea. Avoid rubbing the eyes, so as not to cause further irritation. Use only products that are certified ophthalmological grade.

EYE IRRITATION

see Allergic Reactions

FATIGUE

Fatigue is the second most common complaint doctors hear. Fatigue is more than tiredness; it is an inner feeling of difficulty in performing the most basic physical tasks and usually leads to a *"bad attitude."* It can be caused from serious disorders such as anemia, cancer, chronic viral infections, low thyroid hormone production, hypoglycemia, diabetes, allergies, premenstrual syndrome, and the near-exhaustion phase of stress or emotional crisis. It can also be due to correctable factors such as inadequate sleep, malnutrition, or habitual sedentary lifestyle. Clinical depression is often associated with fatigue. Consult the sections on Allergic Reactions and Anemia in this book.

Suggested Treatment: Faithfully take *The Vitality Pak*, *Cell-Wise*, and *ProVex* or *ProVex-Plus* with each meal. Balance exercise with rest. Identify and avoid possible allergic foods in your diet.

FEVER

A rise in body temperature to 100.4 degrees (2 degrees above normal—the new normal temperature is 98.4) is considered a fever. A portion of the brain known as the hypothalamus measures the temperature of the blood. It stimulates hormones to increase the rate of burning fuel and directs blood flow away from the skin, causing chills. In this way, the body has its own internal thermostat. Bacteria and viruses give off hormone-like substances, known as pyrogens, which trigger the same body reaction. A fever that comes and goes or lasts over two weeks may involve the *"resetting"* of the hypothalamus to a higher temperature. Certain types of cancer and brain tumors can cause this. Scientists now generally agree that a fever, up to a point, is healthy and is the body's attempt to *"burn"* the foreign substance or organism out of the body.

Suggested Treatment: If a fever is less than 103 degrees, drink liquids, including *G'Day Melaleuca Tea*, every 1 to 2 hours and restrict activity. Since fevers tend to reduce appetite, restrict solid food. If a fever is above 103, a tepid (warm to normal skin—about 99 degrees) enema is helpful to bring the temperature down. If the fever is above 105 for more than 2 or 3 hours, emergency measures should be taken to reduce it and prevent brain damage.

Fever may also be reduced using: *Counteract Extra-Strength Pain Reliever; CounterAct PM Pain Reliever Plus Sleep Aid; CounterAct Ibuprofen Pain Reliever and Fever Reducer; CounterAct Cold, Allergy, Sinus Medication; CounterAct Kids Multi-Symptom Cold Plus Cough;* or *CounterAct Kids Pain Reliever and Fever Reducer.*

FEVER BLISTERS

see Cold Sores

FLU

see Influenza

FOOD POISONING

Bacteria can spoil improperly-cared-for food. Bacterial wastes called exotoxins trigger fever, chills, nausea, stomach and muscle aches, diarrhea, headaches, and dizziness. Many people come down with the "*flu*" after eating a picnic lunch on a hot summer day. "*Traveler's Flu*" usually affects entire families. Improperly canned low-acid foods, such as green beans, can grow botulism-producing organisms that are fatal! Shellfish, chicken, chemical food additives, mushrooms, and reheated leftovers are common causes of food poisoning.

Suggested Treatment: When traveling, prevention is assured by eating in restaurants that have a reputation for safety. Avoid foods from street vendors. When in an area where the quality of food is unknown, eat only fruit that can be peeled and avoid raw vegetables and salads made from raw vegetables. Care must also be taken, especially in hot weather, to keep perishables cold. As soon as food poisoning is suspected, induce vomiting to minimize absorption of bacterial exotoxins. Drinking a half cup of warm water containing one teaspoon of salt usually works. If possible, drink one cup of boiled *G'Day Melaleuca Tea* every hour. *This is Fiber?!* should be eaten every few hours to speed bowel transit and hold toxins in the stool. If vomiting or diarrhea persists, dehydration is a concern. Obtain medical care if this condition lasts for more than two days in an adult, or one day in a child.

FOUL TASTE IN MOUTH

The human taste buds are highly developed in some people. Certain food tastes are pleasant to some and not so pleasant to others. Disorders of taste can be caused from sinus infections, reduction in smell due to nasal congestion, smoking, or facial nerve damage. Other conditions causing foul tastes are poor dental hygiene, chemical poisoning, heavy metal poisoning, viral infections, or psychological depression. Reduced taste can be due to zinc deficiency in the diet.

Suggested Treatment: If organic causes for the foul taste cannot be determined, begin a systematic treatment plan of your own. Proper daily dental care with *Classic Tooth Polish*, *Breath-Away Mouthwash,* and *Hot/Cool Shot Mouth Spray* can be very helpful in restoring normal taste. Have regular dental checkups. Take *The Vitality Pak, Cell-Wise,* and *ProVex* or *ProVex-Plus* with each meal. Drink 2 to 4 cups of *G'Day Melaleuca Tea* each day. Avoid being around pesticides and herbicides as well as solvents, paints, or petroleum-based products. If you experience frequent nasal congestion, consult your natural physician for allergy testing.

FROSTBITE

Exposure to freezing temperatures can cause ice crystals to form in and between cells, which causes cell damage. The skin stings, itches, burns, and sometimes turns red and/or numb. Peeling or blistering may occur in 24 to 72 hours. Lifetime sensitivity to temperature may develop.

Suggested Treatment: Frostbite can usually be prevented by protecting the body with warm, dry clothing, paying close attention to the hands and feet. When frostbite is suspected, immediate action must be taken to warm the affected area. Since numbness can be an advanced symptom, care should be taken to not overheat the area. Soaking for 30 minutes in water 100 to 110 degrees Fahrenheit is advisable. Then apply *Pain-A-Trate* to maintain micro-circulation. Repeat the soaking and application of *Pain-A-Trate* every hour for four hours. *Sole to Soul Revitalizing Foot Scrub* and *Revitalizing Foot Lotion* can also be used to cleanse and stimulate improved circulation. Be sure to seek medical advice, in addition to following these conservative measures. The affected body part can become sensitive to cold after one attack and can easily suffer other attacks. Regular exercise and massage can help improve circulation in the area.

FUNGAL INFECTIONS

Several considerations are involved in understanding fungi. These organisms belong to the plant kingdom and are found on all healthy skin. Many infections are caused by opportunistic forms of fungi that take advantage of a person's weakened immune system. As such, fungal infections are common in people receiving x-ray therapy, taking birth control drugs, steroids, or antibiotics, diabetics, burn victims, and people with TB or emphysema. Many infections develop during tropical vacations or military service. Severity can vary from a mild rash on the skin to a fatal overgrowth in the lungs. When the infection is localized, it is more easily treated than if it has invaded a major organ. Because of the many forms of fungal infections, microscopic examination of the affected tissue, hair shaft, or sputum is helpful in making a diagnosis. Fungal infections fail to respond to antibiotics and can successfully be treated with *Melaleuca oil*. Fungal infections have different names depending on the area of the body affected:

Skin (*Tinea corporis*)	—	see Ringworm
Feet (*Tinea pedis*)	—	see Athlete's Foot
Nails (*Tinea ungium*)	—	see Ringworm
Scalp (*Tinea capitis*)	—	see Ringworm
Groin (*Tinea cruris*)	—	see Jock Itch
Beard Area (*Tinea barbae*)	—	see Barber's Itch

FURUNCLES

see Boils

GALLSTONES

Excessive dietary fats, high cholesterol, habitual weight loss diets, drugs that affect the liver, a family history of gallstones, birth control pills, and excessive dietary sugar are most commonly associated with gallstone formation. Dull upper back pain, especially near the right shoulder blade after eating a fatty meal, is the most common symptom of gallstone formation. Sudden nausea with pain in the upper, mid, or right stomach area heralds a gallbladder attack, usually at night after retiring. Chemical analysis of blood and stool samples can determine if conditions for gallstone formation are present.

Suggested Treatment: Prevention is best! Avoid fatty foods, and reduce dietary fat intake to less than 20% of the total calories each day. Eat *This is Fiber?!* bars to keep bile flowing through the bowel. Avoid sugar and sugar-containing foods.

GANGRENE

Caused by bacteria, gangrene is a progressive infection that causes death to the tissues and, if untreated, will require amputation. If caused by the clostridium bacteria, moist gangrene causes blisters, oozing fluid, and putrid odors; thus the term gas gangrene. It also has the symptoms of dry gangrene where the affected area turns black, loses feeling, and has red, inflamed surrounding tissue. Some of the causes of gangrene are bad wounds and infections, reduced blood supply to an extremity, diabetes, frostbite, drug reactions, and swelling from large burns. Warning symptoms include pain in the area when at rest and black, blue, or purple colored skin around the affected area. See the sections on Disinfectants, Diabetes, and Frostbite in this book.

Suggested Treatment: See your natural physician if symptoms are suspicious. Depending upon the location and advanced state of the infection, antibiotic therapy may be ineffective and often fails to stop the disease. If caught in the early stages, soak the body part in a solution of 1 oz. of *Sol-U-Mel* and 4 Tbs. Epsom salts in one gallon of very warm water (106 to 110 degrees) for 20 minutes every 2 hours. The wound should be allowed to drain as much as possible. Keep the area warm, since the tissue usually feels hot and swollen. Apply *T36-C5* or *T40-C3* every 2 hours to the affected part. *Pain-A-Trate* can increase local blood circulation to the area and should be applied immediately after *T36-C5* or *T40-C3*.

GASTRIC ULCERS

Stress, aspirin, or spinal nerve irritation, as well as a poor diet, can lead to ulcers by stimulating the Vagus nerve, which controls production of stomach hydrochloric acid. Some scientists insist that the taking of antacids, while giving temporary relief from stomach acid, in the long run actually elevates production of stomach acid. Statistics show that while antacids are being taken at ever increasing frequency, ulcers continue to be one of the most frequently treated conditions. Starting as indigestion and stomach pain, this condition can lead to referred back pain, anemia, and fatigue if uncorrected. Our high-stress lifestyle appears to be the most contributing factor.

Suggested Treatment: For people who have had ulcers for several years, lifestyle should be closely evaluated. The flavonoids in *ProVex* and *ProVex-Plus* help heal ulcers by reducing histamine secretion and by binding to and protecting connective tissue in mucous membranes of the stomach, so take as directed. Drink 2 to 4 cups of *G'Day Melaleuca Tea* each day. Begin an exercise program. Practice relaxation breaks for 20 minutes each day. For acute attacks, drink one cup of *G'Day Melaleuca Tea* every hour. Eat one half of a *This is Fiber?!* bar every 2 hours between meals. Eat cole slaw or have boiled cabbage every four hours (compound U in cabbage stops production of stomach acid). Avoid alcohol, caffeine, smoking, and rich or fatty foods, as these stimulate the production of stomach acid.

GASTRITIS

Gastritis is an irritation in the stomach and/or small intestine, usually caused by gas. Overeating, eating in a hurry, or eating rich foods late at night are the usual causes. Severe gastritis can trigger pains in the chest which are often mistaken for a heart attack.

Suggested Treatment: Celebrate eating by giving thanks, having soft music and candlelight. Take time between bites to have casual conversation, and quit eating just before you are full. If gastritis is common, in spite of these preventive measures, avoid eating anything 3 hours before bedtime, and avoid drinking anything within 1 hour of bedtime. Have only liquids between meals including *G'Day Melaleuca Tea*. Persistent discomfort should be brought to the attention of your natural physician.

GLOSSITIS

Inflammation of the tongue is a sign of a local irritation, or more often, a disease elsewhere. Local causes can include mechanical trauma from jagged teeth, ill-fitting dentures, or repeated biting during convulsive seizures. Other irritants include alcohol, tobacco, hot foods, and spices, or sensitization to chemicals in toothpaste, mouthwashes, breath fresheners, candy dyes, or dental materials. The most common general cause of glossitis is malnutrition or avitaminosis (a deficiency in specific B vitamins). A few rare disorders produce tongue inflammation but are determined by first ruling out these common causes.

Suggested Treatment: Take *The Vitality Pak* every meal. Also take *ProVex* or *ProVex-Plus* to help reduce inflammation. Stop smoking. Use only safe dental hygiene products such as *Classic Tooth Polish*, *Breath-Away Mouthwash*, and *Exceed Dental Floss*. Drink 2 to 4 cups of *G'Day Melaleuca Tea* per day. Have dental checkups regularly. If congestion exists, use *CounterAct Cold/Sinus/Allergy* as directed.

GOUT

A condition with painful joints of the toes, fingers, or other areas, along with elevated blood uric acid, is typically known as gout. Sharp urate crystals cause physical damage to the cartilage. Once known as a "rich man's disease," gout affects those who are usually overweight and consume alcohol, large quantities of red meat, and rich foods. Have a thorough physical examination performed and begin following the doctor's recommendations.

Suggested Treatment: Start a low stress diet consisting of more vegetables (a *"greens and beans diet"*) and fewer animal products. Take *Replenex Joint Replenishing Complex* to help rebuild damaged cartilage. Eat more fruits and vegetables and fewer animal products. Drink 2 to 4 cups of *G'Day Melaleuca Tea* each day. Apply *Pain-A-Trate* to any affected joints 2 to 4 times each day at first, then each morning and evening until painless mobility is achieved. Take a hot soak with 1 capful *Sol-U-Mel* in 1 quart of water 30 minutes each morning to minimize damage to cartilage.

GUM DISEASE

see Bleeding Gums

HAIR LOSS

One cause of hair loss can be an inherited trait seen in middle-aged men. A receding hairline is caused by an accumulation of male hormones, which alters the natural fats secreted in the scalp and stunts hair growth. The characteristic pattern is thinning and baldness beginning in the front and progressing backward over the head. Research has recently shown that men who begin this pattern in their 20's or early 30's instead of the mid-40's have a greater risk of developing heart disease early in life. Male pattern baldness or slow hair loss due to aging has no known proven treatment. It appears to be nature's conservative desire to reduce unneeded plumage as we get older! We do know that protein metabolism (hair is pure protein) slows down by about one-half after the sixth decade of life. We also know that maximizing our nutrition in youth helps avoid or postpone many genetic weaknesses called inborn errors of metabolism.

In conditions other than male pattern baldness, we find quite an array of causes. Doctors have seen partial hair loss in children who were malnourished; patched hair loss due to heavy metal poisoning such as lead; thinning or splitting and lifeless hair due to harsh chemical hair care products; total body hair loss due to stress; and intermittent hair loss in people experiencing bowel parasitic infections. After giving birth, some women will lose up to one-third of their head hair but will quickly grow it back within a year if properly nourished. There have even been a few cases of head lice and dog and cat flea bites that have produced immune reactions in the scalps of children, causing temporary hair loss. Dandruff sufferers, due to scratching, often have mild to heavy hair loss. See the section on Dandruff in this book. Complicated or unresponsive hair loss should be evaluated by your natural physician.

Suggested Treatment: After ruling out the pathological conditions causing hair loss, many people slow down or stop hair loss when simple steps are taken. A daily scalp massage with *T36-C5* or *Moistursil Problem Skin Lotion* is often helpful. Use *Natural Shampoo* to maintain healthy hair and scalp. Above all else, get adequate nutrition including protein. Take *The Vitality Pak* with each meal. Adequate rest to prevent stress is essential. Include moderate exercise in your daily schedule to keep the pores of the skin clean and skin circulation optimal. Drink *G'Day Melaleuca Tea* on a daily basis.

HALITOSIS

see Body Odor

HARDENING OF THE ARTERIES

see Atherosclerosis

HAY FEVER

Hay fever is one of the most commonly seen conditions. Its seasonal symptoms of tree, weed, and grass pollen hypersensitivity include runny, red, and itching eyes and a runny, stopped-up nose. When possible, avoid exposure to the pollens to which you are allergic. Due to cross-sensitivity, food allergies may reinforce pollen allergies. For example, eating wheat may aggravate a wheat pollen allergy. In that case, avoid eating wheat, oats, rye, and barley from May until August.

Suggested Treatment: The flavonoids in *ProVex* have been shown to have an antihistamine action as well as an anti-allergic action, so take

ProVex or *ProVex-Plus* at the rate of one capsule for every 25 pounds of body weight daily. This can be in addition to your daily *ProVexCV* intake. Each night before retiring, swab each nostril of your nose with a cotton-tipped applicator containing *Moistursil Problem Skin Lotion*. This will reduce the accumulated pollen from the day and moisten dry mucous membranes. Take *CounterAct Cold, Allergy, Sinus Medicine* as directed. Take *The Vitality Pak* each meal to boost your immune system. Drink 2 to 4 cups of *G'Day Melaleuca Tea* each day. See also the section on Allergies.

HEADACHE

There are many types, degrees of severity, and locations of headaches. About 80% of all headaches are due to muscle tension or nerve restriction from stress or injury, which inhibits blood flow out of the brain. These respond well to chiropractic adjustment of the vertebral spine and massage of tense muscles. Allergies, eye strain, sinus or dental infections, viruses, high blood pressure, reduced blood oxygen, low blood sugar, or toxemia (constipation, alcohol, chemical fumes, caffeine addiction, etc.) are other common causes. Brain tumors can also cause slowly developing, continual headaches. Migraine headaches usually are one-sided and can be severe enough to cause nausea and reduced vision. Migraine sufferers get dramatic relief from identifying and eliminating specific sensitized foods from their diet.

Suggested Treatment: For tension headache, a gentle massage for 2 to 5 minutes to the back of the neck, on the temples, and on the sinuses over and under the eyes using *Pain-A-Trate* often relieves local muscles and promotes blood circulation. Take special care to keep *Pain-A-Trate* away from your eyes. Applying a hot moist pack to the back of the neck, temples, or over the eyes afterwards completes the treatment. Most tension headaches are relieved within 10 to 15 minutes with this technique. If symptoms do not improve, keep a log of the frequency, severity, and duration of your headaches and see your natural physician. Remember, do the simple things first!

Begin an exercise program to reduce tension. Take *The Vitality Pak* and *Cell-Wise* with every meal. Drink 2 to 4 cups of *G'Day Melaleuca Tea* each day. Take a *This is Fiber?!* bar to maximize bowel elimination. Take *Sustain* drink between meals to maintain blood sugar. Drink water and get plenty of rest. If congestion exists, use *CounterAct Cold/Sinus/Allergy* as directed. *ProVex*, *ProVex-Plus*, and *ProvexCV* have also been found effective in relieving or reducing migraine headaches. *Luminex* also often reduces the incidence of migraine headaches.

HEAD COLD

see Sinus Congestion

HEAD LICE

see Lice

HEARING DISORDERS

see Deafness

HEART DISEASE

see Cardiovascular Disease

HEART PALPITATIONS

Heartbeats you are aware of are referred to as heart palpitations. They can be a normal response, such as occurs immediately following exercise or when excited. Severe physical stress, anxiety, or an overactive thyroid are common causes of unnatural palpitations. Organic heart disease, such as clogged arteries, enlarged heart, congestive heart failure, or ischemia also cause heart palpitations. Some people notice skipped beats or extra beats of their heart. If a feeling of weakness, light-headedness, or difficulty getting a breath accompanies palpitations, consult your physician without delay. See the section on Allergic Reactions in this book.

Suggested Treatment: Reduce stress! Learn to relax! Take *The Vitality Pak, Cell-Wise,* and *ProVexCV* at each meal. Drink 2 to 4 cups of *G'Day Melaleuca Tea* per day.

HEAT EXHAUSTION

Prolonged exposure to high temperatures may lead to either excessive fluid loss, gradual weakness, anxiety, nausea, excess sweating or failure to sweat, headaches, weakness, or sudden loss of consciousness (heatstroke). Advanced cases of heat exhaustion are emergency situations, requiring immediate cooling of the body to prevent death.

Suggested Treatment: Common sense is the best preventive measure. Strenuous exertion or wearing heavy, insulated clothing in a hot or inadequately ventilated environment should be avoided. Fluids and electrolytes should be replaced by drinking cool (not too cold) *G'Day Melaleuca Tea* or *Sustain* drink every hour. If exposure to heat is prolonged for several days, and heavy perspiration is maintained, *The Vitality Pak* and *Cell-Wise* should be taken with every meal to replace lost minerals and maintain temperature regulation mechanisms within the brain. If conditions are severe, get immediate medical attention.

HEMORRHOIDS

Hemorrhoids are varicosities of the veins of the hemorrhoidal plexus in the anus, often accompanied by inflammation, reddening, and bleeding. Seldom are they painful unless accompanied by more advanced conditions such as fissures (tears) or fistulas (burrow-like tracts from the inner anus to non-healing sores around the anal area). Over 50% of adults are bothered by hemorrhoids. There are Biblical accounts of piles (hemorrhoids). Hemorrhoidal veins contain blood that is not emptying properly into the portal circulation to the liver. Constipation, laxative-induced diarrhea, pregnancy, and occupations requiring long seating on hard or cold objects tend to cause this itching, burning irritation. Constipation causes excess lower bowel pressure and can cause the external hemorrhoid veins to enlarge suddenly. Thin or flat-on-one-sided stool or a full feeling immediately after a bowel movement is a good indication of internal hemorrhoids.

Suggested Treatment: Preventing this condition is best. Get adequate exercise and water each day. Take *ProVex*, *ProVex-Plus*, or *ProVexCV* each day as recommended. A *This is Fiber?!* bar should also be taken every day to prevent constipation. A cotton ball or 2 x 2 inch gauze pad soaked with *T36-C5* or *Pain-A-Trate* held in the anal opening can quickly reduce the itching and burning. *Mela-Gel* applied to the area can also bring quick relief.

Chronic hemorrhoids are best treated as follows. Add 1 oz. of *Sol-U-Mel* and 1 oz. of *Moistursil Bath Oil* to 1 quart of warm water. Sponge the solution onto the hemorrhoidal area. Leave for several minutes. Pat dry. Apply *Mela-Gel*, *Moistursil Problem Skin Lotion*, or *Triple Antibiotic Ointment*. Repeat the procedure morning and night for seven days. A hot sitz bath each evening with the above solution may be very helpful in shrinking any external hemorrhoids. Stubborn hemorrhoids may require conservative therapy beyond the use of Melaleuca products. Contact your natural physician about non-surgical hemorrhoid treatment.

HERPES SIMPLEX

see Cold Sores

HERPES ZOSTER

see Shingles

HICCUPS

Hiccups are repeated involuntary spasms of the diaphragm, followed by sudden closures of the glottis, which stop the inflow of air and produce the characteristic sounds. Some people are more prone to hiccups from drinking alcohol, taking certain medications, or dealing with bladder irritations, excitement, and certain disorders of the stomach or bowel. High blood carbon dioxide seems to reduce hiccups.

Suggested Treatment: Many different treatments have been tried, from the very simple (holding your breath) to the quite extreme (surgically cutting the nerve going to the diaphragm!) The most common do-it-yourself methods that may work are: breathe in and out deeply but slowly into a paper bag (not plastic as it may cling to nostrils); take a series of deep breaths and hold them as long as possible; swallow dry bread, honey or crushed ice; induce vomiting; pull and hold the tongue; put direct finger pressure on your eyeball; drink cool *G'Day Melaleuca Tea* from the far side of a glass by bending your head down between your knees. In spite of all these methods, including surgery and powerful drugs, some cases of hiccups have been recorded to last for weeks.

HIGH BLOOD PRESSURE

No single cause is known for hypertension. Whatever the cause, it will lead to either a restriction of blood flow in the blood vessels or increased heart pumping. Family tendencies are often seen as the most common trait. Lifestyle factors such as type "A" personalities (high stress), smoking, high blood cholesterol and triglycerides, alcohol consumption, and caffeine consumption predominate. Contrary to popular belief, salt consumption in healthy people does not increase blood pressure. (Low blood pressure, however, is often due to a deficiency of salt.) Those who are under high stress and have high blood pressure benefit from restricting salt intake. Actually, deficiencies in many other essential nutrients including magnesium, potassium, and B vitamins are known to be present in people who have high blood pressure, and they are helped by supplementation. See the section on Cardiovascular Disease in this book.

Suggested Treatment: Progressive exercise helps high blood pressure by reducing stress hormones and increasing the efficiency of the vascular system. Take *The Vitality Pak* and *Cell-Wise* with each meal. Take *ProvexCV* to regulate platelet activity and increase vascular integrity. Drink 2 to 4 cups of *G'Day Melaleuca Tea* each day.

HIVES

Hives are a form of skin rash that consists of raised white welts mixed with red patches on the skin. The cause of hives is an allergic or hypersensitive reaction. Drug allergies, severe stress, insect stings or bites, ingestion of certain foods (particularly eggs, shellfish, nuts or fruits), and desensitization injections can cause hives from a hypersensitive reaction. Certain virus infections such as hepatitis, mononucleosis, and measles can be announced by the sudden appearance of hives. Hives lasting two weeks or longer can be due to an allergic reaction to drugs or chemicals such as penicillin in milk, non-prescription drugs, food preservatives, dyes, or other food additives. Hives can also result from animal dander. Determine the source and avoid it in the future.

Suggested Treatment: The flavonoids in *ProVex* have shown to have an antihistamine action as well as an anti-allergic action, so take *ProVex* or *ProVex-Plus* at the therapeutic dose of 1 capsule for every 25 pounds of body weight per day until relief is found. This can be in addition to taking your *ProVexCV* every day as recommended. Application of *T36-C5*, *Mela-Gel*,

Pain-A-Trate, or soaking in a warm bath with 4 oz. of *Sol-U-Mel* and 4 oz. of *Moistursil Bath Oil* usually returns normal circulation to the affected area. Drink *G'Day Melaleuca Tea* 2 to 4 times each day to assist in detoxification. If congestion exists, use *CounterAct Cold, Sinus & Allergy* as directed. Chronic hives can be due to an underlying disease and should be brought to the attention to your natural physician.

HOARSENESS

Hoarseness is due to inflammation of the voice box (larynx) and can be caused from simple overuse, such as yelling at an athletic event, or other disorders such as viral or bacterial infections.

Suggested Treatment: Inhale steam made from adding 10 drops of *T36-C5* and 2 capfuls of *Sol-U-Mel* to the water in a steam vaporizer. Drink hot *G'Day Melaleuca Tea* 2 to 6 times each day. Resting the voice usually reduces the symptoms within a few days and prevents further inflammation. For serious cases, seek medical attention.

HOT FLASHES

Not to be confused with a fever, hot flashes can appear suddenly with a stiflingly stuffy hot feeling and reddened sweaty head, face, and neck skin lasting from a few seconds to several minutes. They are often followed by chills. Hot flashes occur in over 75% of women at menopause and may occur for more than 5 years. Pregnant women may also experience hot flashes. Menopausal-aged women frequently experience these sudden hot spells with profuse perspiration during the day or night. Adrenal-pituitary "storms" create an unstable hypothalamus which brings about inadequate thermal regulation. Insomnia and resulting anxiety can be a complication. Apparently, the hypothalamus of the brain becomes unable to coordinate with other hormone fluctuations and body temperature changes, due to declining estrogen levels. Busy lifestyles and inadequate rest may intensify the general symptoms. Stress also can play a moderate part.

Suggested Treatment: Reduced stress is vital for control of hot flashes. Avoid sugar, caffeine, red meat (arachadonic acid), and chocolate. Use cold pressed olive oil as a salad dressing. Get enough rest (night sleep and mid-day nap) and aerobic exercise. Take *EstrAval* and *Luminex* as directed. Maintain proper nutrition including *The Vitality Pak*, *Cell-Wise*, and *ProVex* or *ProVex-Plus*. Also enjoy 2 to 4 cups of *G'Day Melaleuca Tea* daily.

HOT TUBS

No Melaleuca products, including *T36-C5*, *Moistursil Bath Oil*, or *Sol-U-Mel*, should be used in an operating hot tub or permanent Jacuzzi tub. *Melaleuca alternifolia* oil is not compatible with the filtration system in these sophisticated environments.

HYPERTENSION

see High Blood Pressure

HYPOGLYCEMIA

Low blood sugar accounts for more behavioral symptoms than any single condition. Afternoon fatigue, forgetfulness, dull headaches, multiple food allergies, anti-social behavior, difficulty losing weight, bad dreams, sweet or alcohol cravings, sudden loss of energy, eating disorders, fits of anger or depression, body aches, poor protein digestion and slow physical reflexes are the more common symptoms. Stress, overconsumption of refined sugar, and nutritional deficiencies of minerals and B vitamins appear to be the causes of hypoglycemia. Up to 50% of Americans randomly tested with a 6-hour glucose/insulin tolerance test have an abnormal response. Since the nervous system cannot store fuel, it must constantly be bathed in glucose for normal function. (One judge in California is noted for not granting a divorce to couples until they have both taken a glucose tolerance test.) Children experiencing hyperactive behavior following a sugary holiday are well documented by teachers. In adults, sudden drops in blood sugar or low fasting levels (before breakfast) stimulate instincts to eat something or somebody! Many convicted criminals have a history of sugar abuse. Alcohol is the simplest form of sugar. Untreated hypoglycemia in some people tends to produce adult-type diabetes.

Suggested Treatment: Eat nourishing meals with the insurance of *The Vitality Pak*. Avoid refined sugar, caffeine, and cooked fats. Exercise moderately after eating an *Access Bar*. Take *Sustain* drink between meals to prevent sudden blood sugar drops.

INCONTINENCE

Involuntary loss of urine during the day or night (bedwetting) occurs in the very young and very old. About 3% of children have a congenital defect of the urethra which causes leakage and often requires surgical repair. About 12% of the adult population experiences symptoms as mild as dribbling when laughing, sneezing, lifting, or coughing; it can also be experienced by an urgent desire to void followed by involuntary loss of urine. Stress or urinary tract infections can be the possible cause. Mature men with an enlarged prostate gland can have urinary incontinence or retention. Whatever the cause, loss of control of the urinary sphincter muscles is the result. Back injuries, food allergies, alcoholism, emotional disturbances, and B vitamin deficiencies can also be causes of urinary incontinence.

Suggested Treatment: A simple chiropractic adjustment (lower back or upper cervical) for children who wet the bed may solve the problem. Other children become continent after they stop drinking milk. Some need a good B vitamin supplement added to their diet. *Vita-Bears* or *The Vitality Pak* should be taken with each meal.

Women with urinary infections (less than half have any pain or discomfort) should drink 2 to 6 cups of *G'Day Melaleuca Tea* each day—earlier in the day is better. A series of pelvic tilts, called Kegel exercises, are helpful for women who lose urine when they laugh or cough. For those with a stressful lifestyle, strive for stress reduction through exercise. Men over the age of 40 should have a blood test called a PSA performed regularly. *The Vitality Pak*, *Cell-Wise*, and *ProVex* or *ProVex-Plus* should be taken with each meal along with *ProstAvan* and 2 to 6 cups of *G'Day Melaleuca Tea* each day to protect the prostate in men.

INDIGESTION

Gas, belching, or a bloated feeling are signs of inadequate digestion in the stomach. Eating on the run, inadequate chewing, dilution of digestive juices with copious amounts of liquids, and stress all play a great part in causing indigestion. We now know that, in the long run, many antacids can actually make the problem worse. Malabsorption, ulcers, constipation, and low bowel conditions including hemorrhoids and cancer are seen frequently in people who have a history of indigestion.

Suggested Treatment: Celebrate eating. Sit down. Give thanks. Surround yourself with people you love as often as you can. Savor each bite. Use just enough seasoning to bring out the natural taste. Use *Calmicid* for fast relief of acid indigestion, heartburn, and gas. Take *The Vitality Pak, Cell-Wise,* and *ProVex* or *ProVex-Plus* with each meal. Drink 2 to 4 cups of *G'Day Melaleuca Tea* each day—between or after meals. For more serious digestive problems, consult your natural physician.

INFECTIONS

see Abrasions, Cuts, and Disinfectants

INFLUENZA (FLU)

Influenza is an infectious disease caused by a virus. Its many symptoms may include chills, fever, cough, headache, aches in the joints, weakness, and stomach distress. Much more severe than the common cold, the flu can progress to total exhaustion, acute bronchitis, pneumonia, and sometimes death. Since the virus is spread from one person to another, controlling the environment is important. Keeping one's immune resistance up is the best prevention.

Suggested Treatment: Upon the first signs of the flu, immediately take *Activate Immune Complex* as directed. Start drinking *G'Day Melaleuca Tea* and hot *Sustain* to prevent exhaustion. Use *CounterAct Cough Relief Medicine* as directed. Take *CounterAct Cold, Allergy, Sinus Medicine* as directed. Go to bed. Use *Calmicid Antacid Plus+* if indigestion or gas is present. Begin a steam vaporizer with 10 drops of *T36-C5* and 2 capfuls of *Sol-U-Mel* in the infected person's room. Take *ProVex* or *ProVex-Plus* as directed, and *Cell-Wise* every 2 to 4 hours for the antioxidant effect which reduces pain of muscles, chest, and abdomen.

INGROWN TOENAILS

Ingrown toenails are usually due to poorly fitting shoes. One method of preventing a recurrence is to file a V notch on the middle of the nail so that the point nearly touches the quick. This will cause the nail to draw towards the center and prevent the embedding of the edges of the nail. Trimming in a rounded fashion is not recommended as this actually causes further ingrown toenails. If possible, carefully remove the ingrown part of the nail.

Suggested Treatment: Soak the foot for 15 minutes in a solution of 1 oz. *Sol-U-Mel* per quart of hot water. Dry thoroughly. Apply *T36-C5* followed by *Mela-Gel* or *Triple Antibiotic Ointment*. Repeat morning and night. *Sole to Soul Revitalizing Foot Scrub* and *Revitalizing Foot Lotion* can also be used to cleanse and stimulate improved circulation. If there is an infection, see the section on "Abscesses" in this book.

INSECT BITES

Most plagues and life-threatening communicable diseases have had biting insects (or other families of bugs) as carriers. From the fleas carrying black plague throughout Europe to the malaria-carrying mosquito that took the life of Alexander the Great, insect bites should not be taken lightly. Many unexplained itches and tiny sores on sleepers have been due to nocturnal flying and crawling bugs attracted by body heat. These insects can remain dormant in an unattended dwelling for years awaiting their next (or first) meal.

Suggested Treatment: When staying in a cabin or beach house, immediately fumigate the area with 10 drops of *T36-C5* in a pan of boiling water. The insect repellent properties of Melaleuca oil are international—this works anywhere. Apply *T36-C5* to children's clothing or spray with diluted *Sol-U-Mel* when going to natural parks or walking in the forest in the spring. Mix a few drops *T36-C5* in *Body Satin Hydrating Body Lotion* or *Hand Creme* to spread over the skin.

Inspect your children and yourself daily for small breaks in the skin indicating bites. If you discover an attached "tick" upon your inspection, cover the tick in *T36-C5*. The tick should soon "let go", and you'll be able to remove it easily. Apply *T36-C5*, *Mela-Gel*, or *Triple Antibiotic Ointment* and cover with a bandage for 24 hours.

INSECT STINGS

see Bee and Wasp Stings

INSOMNIA

Insomnia is a condition characterized by the inability of a person to fall asleep or by wakefulness in the middle of the night. Some of the possible causes are a stressful lifestyle, indigestion, over-excitement, pain, discomfort, coffee or other stimulants, or drugs. General good health is the best approach in preventing insomnia.

Suggested Treatment: Avoid caffeine, nicotine, alcohol, sugar, and a sedentary lifestyle. Regular daily exercise, deep breathing, drinking most liquids early in the day, and practicing a philosophy that lives life in one-day segments are good habits to insure good sleep. A relaxing walk after dinner helps digestion and promotes good sleep. Take *Calmicid Antacid Plus+* if heartburn, acid indigestion, or gas are present. Taking *The Vitality Pak* and *Cell-Wise* with each meal and *Sustain* drink while being active will prevent the body from becoming imbalanced in neurohormone production.

ITCHING AND FLAKING SKIN

Itching and flaking skin can be caused by several different health concerns. Those suffering from psoriasis or allergies can experience itchy and flaky skin. This condition may also be seen in people whose diet is deficient in essential oils and some who are post-menopausal. Also see the sections on Allergic Reactions and Psoriasis in this book.

Suggested Treatment: Bathe with *Moistursil Bath Oil*. Wash with *Bath & Shower Gel* or *The Gold Bar*. Apply *Body Satin Hydrating Lotion, Hand Creme*, or *Moistursil Problem Skin Lotion* to troubled areas. Take *ProVex* or *ProVex-Plus* to help restore skin suppleness and elasticity. See your natural physician for further instructions.

ITCHING ANUS

see Pruritis Ani

JOCK ITCH

Fungal infections of the groin, commonly known as jock itch, can form ring lesions around the sides of the crotch. Scratching of the area can cause secondary infections or chronic dermatitis. The lesions may be complicated by a secondary bacteria or yeast such as candida. The occurrences are chronic since the fungus may persist indefinitely or may repeatedly infect susceptible individuals. It occurs more often during the summer or when humidity is high.

Suggested Treatment: Bathing in 1 oz. of *Sol-U-Mel* and using the *Antibacterial Liquid Soap* or *The Gold Bar* is helpful in controlling the fungus. After pat drying, apply *Dermatin Antifungal Creme* as directed. *Mela-Gel*, *T36-C5*, and *Triple Antibiotic Ointment* are also effective. If irritation occurs, or if there is no improvement, discontinue and consult your natural physician.

KIDNEY STONES

Kidney stones can be formed in the kidneys, ureter, bladder, prostate or urethra. Their movement down the urinary tract can produce pain, bleeding, obstruction, and secondary infection. Milk drinkers and those who do not drink enough water tend to make stones from super-saturated urine. Patients who have passed stones describe them as *"a red hot bowling ball with razor blades,"* while others say it is *"ten times worse than having a baby."* One third of a million Americans are hospitalized each year with kidney stones. Some people have had 3 or more surgeries over the years for stones. Modern ultrasound shattering (lithotripsy) is being performed but can damage the kidneys, spleen and lymph nodes as well. Since their formation conforms to the rules of chemistry, they can usually be prevented. About 80% of stones in Americans are composed of calcium salts, about 5% are uric acid, and 2% are made up of the amino acid cystine, with the rest being made up of a mixture of phosphates released during infections or from medications. Many stones are *"silent"* until they begin to move. Some produce back pain or radiating pains into the groin area. Occasionally nausea, chills, fever and abdominal swelling are present.

Suggested Treatment: If there is a family or personal history of stone formation, avoid dairy products completely. Drink plenty of water and 2 to 6 cups of *G'Day Melaleuca Tea* per day. Take *The Vitality Pak, Cell-Wise,* and *ProVex* or *ProVex-Plus* with each meal. Ask your druggist about the side effects of all medications you are prescribed. If back or abdominal pain is present, apply *Pain-A-Trate* to the affected area along with a hot pad. Take a long hot bath. The stone will pass easier if you are relaxed and comfortable.

LARYNGITIS

see Hoarseness

LEG CRAMPS

Leg cramps are due to either a deficiency in circulating calcium or reduced oxygen to muscles. Muscle cramps tend to appear after unconditioned physical activity. Stretching a "crampy" muscle can prevent knotting.

Suggested Treatment: Exercise in three steps: warm up for 5 minutes to stretch muscles, do your work out, then cool down by moving slower or walking until the heart returns to its pre-exercise rate. Eat an *Access Bar* 15 minutes before beginning exercise. Take *The Vitality Pak* with each meal. Drink *G'Day Melaleuca Tea* and *Sustain* before, during, and after exercise to reduce stress on the body. Take *Cell-Wise* with each meal to properly oxygenate muscle cells during exercise without free radical formation. Persons who are bedridden may need the assistance of external pneumatic compression boots to maximize circulation and prevent leg pains. Consult your natural physician.

LEUKOPLAKIA

Leukoplakia are white lesions on the skin inside the mouth. They are occasionally precancerous. While no certain cause is known, suspicion is aimed toward chemical irritations from smoking tobacco, chewing tobacco, food additives, food preservatives, food colorings, and dental materials, as well as toothpastes, mouthwashes, and oral medications that contain alcohol, which tends to dry the mucosa. This condition is seen in people of all ages.

Suggested Treatment: Discontinue contact of questionable substances with the oral mucosa. Use *Classic Tooth Polish*, *Breath-Away Mouthwash*, and *Hot/Cool Shot Mouth Spray*. Drink 2 to 6 cups of *G'Day Melaleuca Tea* daily. Take *The Vitality Pak*, *Cell-Wise*, and *ProVex* or *ProVex-Plus* with each meal.

LICE (see also "Body Lice")

Lice are small parasitic insects that feed on the victim's blood.

Suggested Treatment: Immediately upon suspecting or seeing evidence of lice, shampoo with *Natural Shampoo* and bathe in a mixture of 1 oz of *Sol-U-Mel* and 1 oz of *Moistursil Bath Oil*. Afterward, massage *T36-C5* into scalp and hair to soften and dislodge the nits (the eggs of the lice). Don't be stingy with the oil! Comb the oil through the hair. To fumigate the live insects, wrap your hair in a hot moist towel for 10 minutes. Repeat every second day for at least 5 treatments (10 days). To avoid reinfection, wash all clothing and bedding with *MelaPower* laundry detergent plus *Sol-U-Mel* in hot water. Add 2 ounces of *Sol-U-Mel* to 16 ounces of water and spray the entire house, especially affected areas.

LIVER DISORDERS

The liver is the master chemist of the body. Every bite of food, every ounce of non-food chemicals (Americans ingest more than 11 pounds per year), and every waste product of the cells in the body is processed through the liver. The liver is so vital to life that we have been given one that is seven times larger than needed. Yes, we could actually have six-sevenths removed surgically and still live. The liver would respond by growing to its original size—a feat that no other organ can do. Besides genetic defects, disorders of the liver are classified by two main types—toxic and infectious. Liver toxicity occurs from alcohol consumption as well as storing substances in the liver that are unable to be detoxified. Infectious damage occurs from such conditions as mononucleosis, hepatitis, and parasites. Once the liver is damaged, it begins to affect every other function and system of the body. Protecting the liver is of vital concern in these days of environmental pollution and untreatable infectious diseases.

Suggested Treatment: Drink plenty of purified water. Prepare food in a safe manner and demand safe handling by food establishments. Drink

2 to 4 cups of *G'Day Melaleuca Tea* each day. Take *The Vitality Pak, Cell-Wise, and ProVex* or *ProVex-Plus* with each meal.

NOTE: Allowing the liver to detoxify is essential for health. Our great grandmothers used to give the family sulfur and molasses, along with cod liver oil, each spring. Unless you are a child, pregnant, nursing or hypoglycemic, you may want to do the following spring and fall liver cleanse:

Eat only raw, steamed, or juiced vegetables, or vegetable soup and rice for one week. Drink one quart of apple juice along with 2 to 6 cups of *G'Day Melaleuca Tea* each day. On the sixth and seventh day, take one-fourth to one-half cup of olive oil followed by 1 tablespoon of Epsom salt dissolved in citrus juice. Stay close to home those days. Some nausea may occur due to the release of bile. Contact your natural physician if you have questions.

LONGEVITY

The human body and mind are designed to last one hundred and twenty years. Illnesses, stress, and accidents can shorten that span. Much of our ability to live a full and active life has to do with planning to be well and taking preventive measures against disease early in life. Using health-building Melaleuca products enhances wellness and enjoyment of life. We all will get older, but aging can be slowed significantly using these products.

Suggested Treatment: Drink plenty of purified water. Drink 2 to 4 cups of *G'Day Melaleuca Tea* each day. Take *The Vitality Pak, Cell-Wise,* and *ProVex* or *ProVex-Plus* with each meal. The antioxidants in *Cell-Wise* and *ProVex* products are the best defense available against free radical activity, which causes aging. Use *Access Bars* daily to help burn stored fat and maintain muscle tone. Take *NutraView* daily to prevent macular degeneration and cataracts. Use *Nicole Miller Skin Care* to fight aging of the skin and to maintain healthy skin.

LOW BLOOD SUGAR

see Hypoglycemia

LYME DISEASE

As man invades forests for living space and also wishes to keep things "*natural*," a new ecological balance between man and the environment takes place. Left to themselves, deer, mice, and ticks have gotten along nicely with a parasitic organism called *Borrelia burgdorferi* for a long time. In 1975, a strange illness appeared with symptoms of inflammation and lesions on the skin, followed weeks later with nerve, heart, and joint destruction. Many cases showed up in a rural community near Lyme, Connecticut. Researchers found that the newly discovered parasite needed the mouse and tick to grow on and required the deer for the adult to thrive. Removing any one of these three would stop the spread of the disease. Forty-three states, areas of Europe, China, Japan, and Australia have the disease. The disease in humans starts with a tick bite causing a red macule or papule (usually on the thigh, buttock or under the arm) that grows over a few weeks up to 10 inches across then slowly disappears leaving the chronic symptoms. See the section on Insect Bites in this book.

Suggested Treatment: Prevention is the best way to deal with this condition. A few drops of *T36-C5* mixed with Melaleuca *Hand Creme* makes an effective insect repellent. Diluted *Sol-U-Mel* is also effective. If a tick bite is suspected, apply *T36-C5* every 4 hours until irritation subsides. *Triple Antibiotic Ointment* and *Mela-Gel* should be applied morning and evening under a bandage. For further assistance, contact your natural physician.

MACULAR DEGENERATION

Macular degeneration is the deterioration of the central focal region of the back of the eye called the macula, resulting in impaired vision. The symptoms can be gradual or sudden, with objects usually appearing distorted in one eye. Upon examination, degeneration is often found in the normal appearing eye as well. Both men and women, mostly elderly, contract this condition and seldom have any other eye problems. There may be a hereditary link. Since the condition involves lack of nurturing of this normally blood-rich tissue, some scientists believe it is similar to brain tissue degeneration taking place in senility and atherosclerosis. See the sections on Atherosclerosis and Cardiovascular Disease in this book. Laser treatments are often used to treat advanced cases.

Suggested Treatment: Take *NutraView*, which promotes long-term macular health and visual acuity with lutein, bilberry, blueberry, and Vitamin C. Take *The Vitality Pak* and *Cell-Wise* with each meal. Take *ProVex-Plus* daily to promote vascular integrity. Drink 2 to 4 cups of *G'Day Melaleuca Tea* each day. If you are older than 60, get a visual field evaluation test performed by your eye doctor every year.

MASSAGE

One of the oldest and most widely practiced health-preserving therapies known is massage (see Bathing). Part of its benefits are the mechanical effect of "*rubbing*" and "*kneading*" tensions from the body. Many times we are unaware of these tensions until we are actually being massaged. Often, we can massage certain muscles on our own bodies. However, the greatest benefit is often received when it is done by a trained pair of gentle hands. There are several different techniques, each having certain advantages in specific situations. Massage is especially recommended for those who are bedridden or who are unable to exercise. Well-muscled people can usually withstand more vigorous techniques, while those with less muscle will be comfortable with more gentle techniques. Modern massage therapists are trained in multiple techniques to meet your level of need and comfort.

Suggested Treatment: Start by taking a hot bath with 1 to 2 oz. of *Moistursil Bath Oil* for 20 to 30 minutes. Feel the smoothness of your skin. The person receiving the massage must be in a comfortable position, usually face down. The person giving the massage must not feel hurried or uncomfortable when bending at the waist. Apply ample amounts of warmed *Body Satin Lotion* to one extremity, neck, upper back, or lower back area at a time. Rub *Pain-A-Trate* into tender muscles and over stiff or painful joints. A few drops of *T36-C5* can be massaged into areas that feel cold and need better circulation. Massage the limbs toward the heart area, not away from the center of the body. When done gently, you can do no harm.

MEASLES

Rubeola, also known as red measles, is a highly contagious viral infection characterized by fever, bronchial cough, sneezing, and irritated eyes that are sensitive to light. A brownish-red rash starts around the ears, on the face and neck, then spreads over the trunk and occasionally the limbs; it usually lasts 4 to 7 days. Incubation is 7 to 14 days. It is easily transmitted from 2 to 4 days before the rash appears, and from 2 to 5 days after the rash disappears. In most cases, a person only has the measles once. Some people who are weakened by the measles suffer complications such as lung or middle ear infections. Also see "Rubella" in this book.

Suggested Treatment: In well-nourished children and adults, measles usually passes without complications. In malnourished or unhealthy individuals, great care must be taken to prevent a weakened immune system. Preventing ear infections (see Ear Infections), bacterial infections (see Disinfectants), and pneumonia is a primary goal. To prevent respiratory complications, use a warm steam vaporizer in the person's room with 10 drops *T36-C5* and 2 capfuls *Sol-U-Mel*. Drink *G'Day Melaleuca Tea* 3 to 6 times each day.

MENOPAUSE

The change of life for a woman should be celebrated with her husband one year after her last menses. This marks the end of child bearing and the beginning of mentoring of younger women. Menopause (stopping of flow) may be natural (average age 45 to 51), artificial (radiation or surgery) or premature (illness or stress induced). In a state of health, natural menopause has mild symptoms as the ovaries cease producing eggs and shrivel up like gray-colored prunes. When a woman undergoes premature menopause, there are underlying causes that need specific attention. The greatest concern during and for about 5 years after menopause is the rapidly dwindling levels of estrogen to the cells of the body. Various lifestyle factors can have a great effect on estrogen production at this time of life, including stress vs. rest cycles.

Hot flashes (see Hot Flashes), sweating, or light headedness affects about 75% of menopausal women and lasts for about a year. About 25 to 50% of these women have these symptoms for about 5 years or more. Other symptoms of tiredness, weight gain, headaches, irritability, insomnia, and nervousness may be related to both estrogen deprivation and the stress of aging and changing lifestyle roles. Lack of sleep due to disturbances from hot flashes makes the fatigue and irritability worse. Occasional dizziness, numb or tingling sensations, palpitations, and fast heart rate may occur. The risk of heart disease increases. Urinary incontinence and urinary tract infections increase. Nausea, low bowel gas, constipation or diarrhea, and joint and muscle pains are also common complaints. The major health risk is osteoporosis (see Osteoporosis) at this time. Preventing this problem should be every woman's primary health concern now.

Suggested Treatment: See your natural physician and begin following his advice for controlling stress. Take *EstrAval Natural Support for Menopause* daily as directed. Take *The Vitality Pak, Cell-Wise* with each meal, and *ProvexCV* as directed. Begin a daily exercise program using the *Access Bar* and *Sustain* drink to prevent low blood sugar and fatigue. Drink 2 to 4 cups of *G'Day Melaleuca Tea* each day to prevent urinary tract infections. Communication is very important during this time. Overwork and continued stress can prolong symptoms.

MENSTRUAL PAIN

see Cramps

MIGRAINE HEADACHES

see Headache

MONONUCLEOSIS

The presence of fatigue, fever, sore throat, and enlarged lymph nodes signifies the illness known as "*Mono*" which is caused by the Epstein-Barr virus. About 50% of children contact the virus before the age of five and have mild or no symptoms. Recovery is rapid. When infection occurs in young adults, an immune system battle results, where damage is done to human lymphocytes, the spleen, and the liver. Relapses are common if activity is resumed too soon. Many high school and college students miss school because of not heeding the necessary "*rest-and-recover*" treatment. No medicines are known to treat this illness.

The incubation time of the virus is not fully known, but one week to two months is common. The illness can take up to three months to run its course. Complications can occur if it is not properly treated. "*Mono*" can go on to cause seizures, meningitis, psychosis, chronic fatigue syndrome, respiratory disease, jaundice, and hepatitis. Blood testing can detect past infections for several years after the illness has passed.

Suggested Treatment: Complete bed rest for the first several weeks is often necessary to ease symptoms and prevent complications. Mild activity with mid-day rest periods is recommended for the first 4 to 6 weeks. Drink 2 to 6 cups of *G'Day Melaleuca Tea* each day. Take *The Vitality Pak, Cell-Wise,* and *ProVex* or *ProVex-Plus* with juice or broth for the first 2 to 3 weeks, then with meals. Breathe *T36-C5* enriched steam vapor to prevent respiratory complications. Hot baths with 1 oz of *Sol-U-Mel* and 1 oz. of *Moistursil Bath Oil* for 30 minutes are helpful in the absence of a fever. Do not do heavy lifting, bending at the waist, or jumping for 3 months as permanent damage to the liver or spleen may occur.

MORNING SICKNESS

On about the tenth day after conception, the developing placenta begins producing the hormones HCG and estrogen, which may cause mild to severe nausea and vomiting in susceptible mothers-to-be. This, along with tender breasts and no menstrual period, is strong (but not absolute) evidence of pregnancy. A self-administered pregnancy test can be performed on urine, and they are now sensitive enough to be accurate only a few days after conception.

Suggested Treatment: There are no FDA approved drugs for morning sickness. Any anti-nausea drugs can cause damage to the developing baby. Drink and eat small amounts of bland foods (steamed vegetables, baked potato, dry bread, etc.) throughout the day to not stretch the stomach and trigger the very sensitive gag reflex. The first food and drink should be before getting out of bed in the morning. *Sustain* drink is a helpful supplement at this time. Small amounts of *G'Day Melaleuca Tea* taken throughout the day are very calming to the stomach. The need for vitamin B6 and magnesium is great and can be supplied from *The Vitality Pak Prenatal* (they may need to be ground up and put in a drink or taken in the middle of the night). Ginger is a very good herb for controlling nausea and has no side effects. The use of wrist straps fitted with acupressure beads help some women with morning sickness.

MOUTH ULCERS

see Canker Sores

MUCOUS

Thin, watery mucous is a product of healthy membranes in the body and is needed to protect soft tissues from damaging environmental substances. Thick, discolored or stringy sputum (phlegm), and vaginal, eye, stool, or nasal mucous are signs of irritation or infection. Mild bacterial growth, viruses, chronic yeast or fungal infections, digestive problems, stress, allergies and chemical sensitivities can produce this type of mucous.

Suggested Treatment: Drink 2 to 6 cups of *G'Day Melaleuca Tea* each day to reduce the number of harmful organisms in the bowel and urinary tract. Use *CounterAct Cough Relief Medicine* as directed. Take *CounterAct Cold, Allergy, Sinus Medicine* as directed. Breathe steam inhalation with *T36-C5* to clear tear ducts, nasal, and sinus mucous membranes. Douche with *Nature's Cleanse* as directed to reduce vaginal viruses, yeast, molds, fungus, and bacteria. Repeat any of the above to maintain healthy mucous.

MUSCLE CRAMPS

see Cramps or Leg Cramps

MUSCLE PAIN

see Athletic Injuries

MUSCLE SPASMS

see Athletic Injuries

MUSCLE STRAIN

There are several levels of muscle strain. Mild strain occurs regularly with all forms of exercise. Severe muscle strains can cause tearing and bruising. Overused muscles, tendons (connecting muscles to bones), and ligaments (connecting bones to other bones) are helped by immediately applying ice to prevent swelling. Keep the ice on for 5 to 10 minutes each hour, until the swelling is reduced.

Suggested Treatment: *Pain-A-Trate* gives dramatic relief from athletic strains. Soaking in a hot bath with *Moistursil Bath Oil* is very relaxing for aching muscles. Shower with *Kiwi Lime Bath & Shower Gel* which contains arnica, a very effective pain reliever.

NASAL CONGESTION

see Sinus Congestion

NAUSEA

The unpleasant feeling that one is about to vomit is part of a regulatory mechanism that allows for expulsion of potentially harmful substances. Nausea is often associated with improper body functions including constipation or gall bladder congestion. It can also be due to such conditions as pregnancy, the flu, bad food, some drugs, confusion of the balance mechanism of the middle ear by irregular motion, a ruptured inner ear membrane, or spinal nerve irritation from vertebral misalignment. Vomiting is the forceful expulsion of the stomach contents produced from involuntary contraction of abdominal muscles. Psychological factors such as "*distasteful*" food can cause nausea with vomiting. Physical stress such as running too fast, children throwing temper tantrums, or strong coughing can induce vomiting. See the sections on Constipation and Indigestion in this book.

Suggested Treatment: Determine the cause. People can get nauseated after taking their supplements either at or between meals. Food in the stomach helps to mix the contents of the tablets so they do not concentrate nutrients on the nerve-sensitive mucosal lining of the stomach. Contact your natural physician if medical advice is needed.

G'Day Melaleuca Herbal Tea can be effective to reduce nausea.

NECK PAIN

see Athletic Injuries and Stiff Neck

NERVOUSNESS

"A sound mind in a sound body" was the Greek ideal for a healthy person. We now know that what impairs one part of our being will affect the other. Nervousness (mild anxiety) can be due to worry about an unfounded or unlikely situation or event. Deprivation of sleep, clinical depression, and the aches and pains that often accompany tense muscles are typical with nervous people. Nervousness tends to be a learned behavior that depletes the body of valuable nutrients, which in turn perpetuates the condition. Chemical addictions, including nicotine (nervous stimulant) and alcohol (nervous depressant), as well as long term prescription drugs, should be avoided and corrected before permanent improvement can take place. A healthy body makes its own chemicals for awareness and response to real problems. It is one way the body responds to stress. Nearly all mental disorders include nervousness as a component of the diagnosis. See the section on Exercise in this book.

Suggested Treatment: See your natural physician and follow his recommendations for stress control, exercise, and diet. Take *Luminex* which contains St. John's wort, Griffonia seed, folic acid and B-12, daily as directed. Take *The Vitality Pak, Cell-Wise,* and *ProVex* or *ProVex-Plus* with each meal. Drink 2 to 4 cups of *G'Day Melaleuca Tea* each day. Practice relaxation and breathing exercises each day. Believe that you can train your body, with help, to be less nervous.

NICOTINE WITHDRAWAL

We are often asked, *"How can I quit smoking?"* The answer is different for each individual. Some people make up their mind to quit and have no symptoms of withdrawal. Others have neurological and psychological symptoms typical of drug addiction. Depression, anxiety, and behavioral changes are common. Since nicotine is of the alkaloid family, along with morphine and codeine, chemical detoxification and needed emotional support are important to recovery. The appetite suppressive effects of nicotine are well known. Compulsive eating during recovery must be compensated for with exercise and adequate nutrition.

Suggested Treatment: See your natural physician and begin following his advice. Take *The Vitality Pak* and *Cell-Wise* with each meal, and *ProVexCV* as directed. Drink 2 to 4 cups of *G'Day Melaleuca Tea* each day. Eat one *This is Fiber?!* bar each day to speed detoxification. Exercise and drink plenty of water. If needed, do not hesitate to get professional guidance. If congestion exists, use *CounterAct Cold, Allergy, Sinus Medicine* as directed.

NUTRITION

Nutrition is more than just getting enough food. It is getting enough of the right food at the right time for the prevailing needs of the body. It is the miracle the body performs when changing the molecular structure of food into living human tissue. Everyone has slightly different needs for nutrition based upon genetics, lifestyle, temperament, geographic location, past illnesses, digestive and absorptive capacity, and stress effects. The best thing you can do (after choosing the right parents) is to determine your unique nutritional needs. Waiting until you have a health problem before getting concerned about nutrition is like waiting until your car engine runs out of oil to become interested in engine lubrication. Just Do It!

Not getting enough food is called malnutrition. On the average, Americans are overfed and undernourished. Choosing "*brands*" that are heavily advertised in place of foods in their original state is often due to clever marketing and advertising techniques. An example is potato chips in place of a baked potato.

Why is the topic of nutrition so important to us? The Surgeon General's Report in 1990 disclosed that "... *eighty percent of all current diseases are due to chronic degenerative states in the body either directly or indirectly related to diet and nutrition.*" Twenty-five years ago, in spite of volumes of published clinical studies, medical scientists lacked "*conclusive*" evidence that heart disease and cancer (number 1 and 2 leading causes of death) were related to diet. More recently, only a few physicians would deny that diet and nutrition are the leading cause and the best prevention for these conditions. This sudden awakening of the public to the "*new*" nutrition has paved the way for fad diets, quick vitamin cures, and overnight experts who have had little training and often less experience in using nutrition as "*the*" first medicine of choice. As Hippocrates said, "*Let your medicine be your food and let your food be your medicine.*" This should not be too difficult to understand.

Suggested Treatment: Consult your natural physician. Learn where your weaknesses are and design a plan to prevent illness. Take *The Vitality Pak, Cell-Wise,* and *ProVex* or *ProVex-Plus* with each meal, or *ProVexCV* as directed. Drink *G'Day Melaleuca Tea* daily. Get enough rest. Learn how to relax. Practice playful activities (those that make you talk, laugh and breathe deeply) every day. The desire for self-nurturing exists when body, mind and spirit are healthy. Some people may need a little help to get started.

OBESITY

The underlying causes of clinical obesity (being more than 20 per cent above your optimum weight, or having more than 40 per cent of your body weight as fat) often stem from boredom eating, stressful eating, childhood or sexual abuse, drug effects, or dysnutrition. See the section on Nutrition in this book. Less than 10% of the cases of obesity seen involve glandular conditions. The obvious problem is in storing more calories than are being burned through metabolic needs and exercise. All chronic degenerative diseases are accelerated when obesity is present.

Our ancestors earned and burned about 4,000 to 6,000 calories each day just in living, working and walking to school. Because of our automated lifestyle, we earn and burn between 1,200 and 2,000 calories each day. Our nutrient needs for vitamins, minerals and cofactors common to food remain the same. What is wrong with this picture?

Many people have lost hundreds of pounds over the years only to gain it right back. This is due to a physiological condition called *"set point."* The hypothalamus gland in the brain constantly monitors the temperature of the inside of the body compared with the outside surface of the body. The appetite center, also located in the hypothalamus, is activated when factors begin to lower blood sugar. Our bodies are then conditioned or *"set"* to burn less when apparent reserves begin to drop. We actually slow down our rate of calorie burning to conserve fuel. This is why people can go on a water diet for a week and not lose more than one or two pounds. Fatigue is the most common complaint when total calories are restricted. What must happen is to change the set point so that the body is satisfied with less intake while it is burning more of its reserves. Restricting dietary fats to less than 20% of daily intake decreases free radicals and hunger sensations. Continuing exercise establishes a new set point which is the permanent way to control weight. See the section on Exercise in this book.

Suggested Treatment: See your natural physician and begin following his advice. Eat an *Access Bar* 15 minutes before exercise. This will allow your body to actually burn stored fat. Plan your meals ahead of time. Remove all unhealthy snack foods from your home. Enjoy *Attain* as a healthy meal replacement. It is especially effective for weight loss when it is mixed with water or rice milk.

Use exercise, instead of eating, as a means of handling stress. If childhood stresses are present to *"any"* extent, contact Overeaters Anonymous and get involved. This non-profit group is an excellent source of free support. If necessary, see a counselor or a natural physician for appetite suppressive herbs, acupuncture, or specific metabolic testing. Seeking help in getting started is far better than reading a HOW TO book and doing it alone. They don't work for 99% the of people who buy them. The weight simply slips back, with interest!

OSGOOD-SCHLATTER'S DISEASE

Young athletes have muscles that are stronger than the actual bone to which they are attached. Heavy track and field events, especially broad jumping, put unusual strain on the thigh muscles as they connect with the tibia just below the knee. Some young athletes develop this crippling disorder due to an avulsion (fracture) which tears away soft bone with pain and swelling of the area. This pain was once called "*growing pains.*" Knee supports are often used to prevent injuries to 14 thru 18 year-olds.

Suggested Treatment: Apply an ice pack for 5 to 10 minutes to acute pain areas. Take *Mela-Cal* with each meal, as well as before and after exercise to maximize bone development. Take *Mel-Vita* with each meal to enhance growth and healing of injuries. Take *ProVex* or *ProVex-Plus* to reduce pain and inflammation. Apply *Pain-A-Trate* directly to the affected area before and after exercise to minimize swelling and pain. Rub exercised thigh muscles with *Pain-A-Trate* to relax tension and stimulate circulation. Jacuzzi or whirlpool massage is excellent for reducing tension. Do not over-train. You have a long life ahead of you.

OSTEOARTHRITIS (see also Arthritis)

A degeneration of joint material including cartilage and bone takes place when complex systems of mechanical injury, biological stress, biochemical irritation, and enzymatic or nutritional deficiencies are upset. There is no single cause for osteoarthritis. Healthy joints have such little friction that without some precipitating condition, they will never wear out. Apparently the amount of friction in the joint increases after repetitive injury (plucking chickens), taking drugs for other conditions (many drugs affect joint and bone metabolism), toxic reactions to environmental pollution (pesticides, herbicides, food additives, etc.), trace nutrient deficiencies, or dietary habits that promote nutritional deficiencies (excessive coffee drinking, alcohol, limited diet selection, etc.). Osteoarthritic joints have less flexible cartilage and more infiltrated bone causing the tell-tale enlarged joints on fingers. Exercise tends to pump nutrients in and wastes out of healthy cartilage. See the section on Arthritis in this book.

Suggested Treatment: Exercise and movement are imperative. Some people who have complained of painful hands, especially in cold weather, have found relief by taking up knitting. Start each morning by doing the evening snack dishes by hand in hot water. Apply *Pain-A-Trate* to the affected joints. Take *Replenex Joint Replenishing Complex* daily for cartilage growth. Take *ProVex* or *ProVex-Plus* to help reduce inflammation. Take *The Vitality Pak* and *Cell-Wise* with each meal. Drink 2 to 4 cups of *G'Day Melaleuca Tea* each day. Consult your natural physician.

OSTEOPOROSIS

There are two major types of osteoporosis, primary and secondary. The primary type occurs more often in women and progresses with age. Known as the *"shrinking disease"*, it affects more women over the age of 65 than breast and uterine cancer combined. The loss of calcium prematurely is due to a combination of factors. Women who are of slight build, smoke cigarettes, consume caffeine and animal products, fail to exercise, and do not ingest enough usable calcium from vegetable sources are prone to develop fractures of large weight bearing bones after menopause. The spine, pelvis, and femoral hip joint areas are most often affected. School-aged girls are often deficient in dietary calcium from vegetable sources. Most are at great risk of never attaining 100% of their expected bone calcium density. Since the expected life span of a woman born in the 1990's is 90+ years, more emphasis should be placed on teaching girls how to prevent this disease.

Secondary osteoporosis is less common and can be due to malabsorption of calcium, endocrine imbalances, prescription or other drug reactions, liver disease, or kidney disease. If you are having any of these problems, consult your natural physician for specific advice.

Suggested Treatment: See your natural physician and begin following his advice. Limit or eliminate all dairy and other animal products. Also eliminate soda pop from your diet. If you are a woman of menopausal age and have lost 1/2 inch or more height since you were 18, begin a program to minimize osteoporosis. If more than 1 inch of height has been lost, consult your natural physician for a calcium metabolism evaluation.

Women of all ages can benefit from taking *EstrAval* daily as directed. Take *The Vitality Pak* and *Cell-Wise* with each meal to insure adequate trace nutrients. Drink 2 to 4 cups of *G'Day Melaleuca Tea* each day to detoxify. Take *ProVex* or *ProVex-Plus* daily. The ingredients in the *ProVex* products are powerful stabilizers of collagen structures, which is the major protein structure in bone.

OTITIS

see Ear Infections

PARONYCHIA

Paronychia is an infection of the tissues around a fingernail or toenail. It is caused by yeast such as *Candida albicans* or bacteria such as *Pseudomonas* or *Proteus*. It enters through a break in the skin. The infection may follow the nail margin and may extend beneath the nail where the infection penetrates more deeply into the finger or toe. Tissue breakdown into the tendons and muscle in the finger or toe may result. Eventually the infected nail may become distorted and lose normal function if not treated promptly.

Suggested Treatment: Early detection and treatment is important. Wash the affected area with *Antibacterial Liquid Soap* and soak for 15 minutes in 1 quart of warm water and 1 oz. of *Sol-U-Mel*. Pat dry. Apply *T36-C5* to the fingernail or toenail morning and night, then follow with *Triple Antibiotic Ointment* or *Mela-Gel*. Cover the area with a loose bandage. Chronic infections may require repeated applications for several months. If *Candida albicans* is the causative agent in a female, douching with *Nature's Cleanse* may be needed to reduce the fungus. Drink *G'Day Melaleuca Tea* 2 to 4 times each day.

PEPTIC ULCERS

see Gastric Ulcers

PHARYNGITIS

see Hoarseness

PIERCED EARS

see Abscesses

PIMPLES

see Acne

POISON IVY, POISON OAK, POISON SUMAC

Complex chemical agents in certain plants are capable of producing acute dermatitis in sensitized individuals. Poison ivy, poison oak, or sumac's blistery rash is a result of coming in contact with the plant itself, or handling the clothing of someone who has been in contact with it. Some people are more sensitive to the oily plant juices than others. Many substances other than poison oak, poison ivy, or sumac cause this acute reaction, including ragweed and primrose. Shoe dyes, formaldehyde in clothing, penicillin, sulfonamides, neomycin, anesthetics, food stabilizers, and cosmetics can also produce severe dermatitis.

Suggested Treatment: Immediate removal of the affecting agent is necessary for any treatment to be effective. Immediately wash the area thoroughly with *Antibacterial Liquid Soap* and warm water. Pat (don't rub) dry. Apply *Triple Antibiotic Ointment* and cover with a loose gauze bandage three times each day until resolved. If the rash or blistering has appeared before treatment can be started, soak gauze bandages in cool *G'Day Melaleuca Tea* and cover the affected area. Re-soak gauze and apply every 15 minutes until pain subsides. Apply *Triple Antibiotic Ointment* three times each day until resolved. Draining the blisters can be done, but do not remove the covering skin. If pain does not reduce, apply *Pain-A-Trate*. Contact your natural physician if improvement is not seen after 4 days.

POLYPS

This is a clinical term which refers to any mass of tissue that protrudes from a mucous membrane in the nose, throat, vocal chord, ear, bowel, vagina, or urinary tract tissue, and extends outward. It may be normal tissue or diseased. While there is no known cause of polyps, reactions to certain drugs, pollutants, or irritants seem linked. Most cancers of the bowel start from a polyp. (Rectal screening by your natural physician should be performed as part of your annual physical examination if you are over 50 years old.)

Suggested Treatment: Bleeding polyps should be seen by your natural physician. Only easily accessed polyps can be treated at home. Apply *Mela-Gel, Triple Antibiotic Ointment,* or *Moistursil Problem Skin Lotion* three times each day for 14 days to polyps. If reduction does not occur, see your natural physician.

PREGNANCY

Pregnancy is a natural process, yet one out of every eleven pregnancies produces an abnormal baby. The best thing to do to have a healthy happy baby is to have healthy, happy parents. External factors that are known to greatly affect a normal pregnancy include the nutrition of the mother and the safety of the environment. Exercise should be continued during pregnancy to maintain muscle tone and prevent back problems from the added 20 to 30 pounds of normal weight gain.

Since the baby is made from molecular building blocks, maximizing nutritional needs and minimizing non-nutritional chemicals is vital. Nutritional needs of the expectant mother increase for all of the known nutrients. A lack of folic acid is now known to cause spinal cord defects in babies of deficient mothers. It is estimated that 85% to 90% of all pregnant women take prescription or over-the-counter drugs during their pregnancy, with 3% to 12% of abnormal pregnancies resulting from their side effects. Drugs and babies do not mix well. Other dangerous substances include carbon monoxide from cigarette smoke, alcohol, and fumes from paint or toxic household cleaners. Actually, common sense gives us good direction in avoiding these things. The heightened sense of smell and taste during pregnancy gives a woman a great defense for her baby. See the sections on Nausea or Morning Sickness in this book.

Suggested Treatment: Plan for your baby at least one year before you intend to get pregnant. Begin taking *The Vitality Pak Prenatal* with every meal. See your natural physician and follow his advice. Exercise for 30 minutes daily—walking is the best prior to the birth of the baby. *The Vitality Pak Prenatal* satisfies all of the minimum recommendations for 18 vitamins and minerals, including folate, during pregnancy. Eating low on the food pyramid automatically gives adequate roughage to prevent constipation and water retention. Toxemia during pregnancy is best prevented by minimizing stress while balancing activity with rest.

PRURITIS ANI

Pruritis Ani is Latin for *"Itching Anus"*. This area of the body tends to have an almost built-in *"readiness to itch."* Itching around the anus can be caused from something as simple as pin worms in children, or as complicated as rectal cancer in adults. Internal hemorrhoids are often discovered as a cause in adults. Many causes stem from chemical irritation with perfumed soap or toilet tissue. Food allergies (particularly eggs or milk) are frequently associated with this condition and often produce a red ring around the anal opening. Food additive sensitivities (colorings, flavorings, and preservatives) are among the most common in children. Other causes include fungal growths such as *Candida albicans*, psychological responses in anxiety patients, other skin problems such as psoriasis or contact dermatitis, heavy coffee or cola drinking, poor hygiene, and over meticulous cleaning with soaps and perfumed powders.

Suggested Treatment: Try to treat the cause. Soaking in a warm bath with 1 cup of Epsom salt and 1 oz. of *Moistursil Bath Oil* often reduces anal muscle tightness which contributes to the itch. Avoid applying or consuming chemical conditioned substances. Drink 2 to 6 cups of *G'Day Tea* each day. Take *The Vitality Pak, Cell-Wise,* and *ProVex* or *ProVex-Plus* with each meal. *Pain-A-Trate* can be dabbed around the anus during extreme cases to minimize itching. *Moistursil Problem Skin Lotion* often gives lasting relief from pruritus ani while the true cause is being corrected. If itching persists, consult your natural physician for further evaluation.

PSORIASIS

Psoriasis is a chronic and recurrent disease of the skin that is characterized by dry, well-circumscribed silvery scaling patches of various sizes. The patches can vary in severity from one or two lesions to a widespread dermatosis with disabling arthritis. The cause is unknown, but it appears to be related to inadequate detoxification possibly through the kidney or the alimentary tract. Thick scaling is probably due to an increased rate of epidermal cell growth. This cosmetic deformity proves socially embarrassing although it is not contagious.

Psoriasis usually involves the scalp and the upper surface of the extremities, particularly the elbows and knees, the back and the buttocks. The nails, eyebrows, armpits, and abdomen or groin region may also be affected. Occasionally the illness is generalized. The lesions are more sharply localized and usually heal without scarring. Hair growth does not appear to be affected. Extension of lesions sometimes produces large plaques up to one-half of an inch thick. Nail involvement may resemble fungal infections, causing a separation of the nail with thickening, discoloration, and debris under the nail plate. Quite often, allergies, stress, and environmental sensitivities should be evaluated. Nutritional needs tend to be elevated during this time.

Suggested Treatment: Bathe using *Antibacterial Liquid Soap* and soak in *Moistursil Bath Oil* for 30 minutes each night. Pat dry (don't rub). Apply *Moistursil Problem Skin Lotion* to the scaly areas. Apply *T36-C5* to newly inflamed or red areas. Cover with *Mela-Gel*. Daily sunlight exposure for 15 to 20 minutes is helpful. Practice relaxation. Eat healthy food. Take *The Vitality Pak, Cell-Wise,* and *ProVex* or *ProVex-Plus* with each meal and drink 2 to 6 cups of *G'Day Melaleuca Tea* daily to help detoxify. Consult your natural physician for further advice.

RASHES

Rashes can be caused by many things. They should be treated to prevent secondary infections and reduce any stinging or itching. See the section on Dermatitis in this book.

Suggested Treatment: Take a hot bath with 1 oz. *Moistursil Bath Oil*, plus 1 oz. *Sol-U-Mel*, and soak for 20 to 30 minutes. Pat dry. Apply *Moistursil Problem Skin Lotion*, *Triple Antibiotic Ointment*, or *Pain-A-Trate* to the affected area. One Air Force officer had suffered 23 years with an extensive body rash he brought back from Viet Nam. He found that the *Problem Skin Lotion* gave him the most symptomatic relief during his slow recovery. He had been burned and poisoned from powerful prescription medications for years and had given up hope, scratching himself to sleep many a night in agony. He now praises these products to everyone he meets—rash free!

RINGWORM

A round, reddened, often bulls-eye appearing rash anywhere on the skin is evidence of ringworm. This superficial infection is caused by dermatophytes fungus (those that invade only dead tissue of the skin, nails, or hair). At least three different strains of fungi can cause ringworm. Household pets such as cats and dogs carry these fungi on their fur and skin. Some cases produce only mild inflammation and often go unnoticed and untreated, then gradually reappear in hot weather. Other types cause a sudden outbreak of a violent-looking rash with vesicles and swelling of the tissue due to a strong immunological reaction of the body against the fungi. Severe itching, especially in the groin area (see Jock Itch), provokes scratching, which tends to spread the infection by the fingernails or causes skin damage and produces secondary infection from bacteria. Since differentiation of these types of fungi is difficult, these infections are approached according to the sites involved. Confirming a diagnosis is made by seeing your natural physician who will scrape a sample of the skin and either examine it under a microscope or send it to the lab for culture.

Suggested Treatment: As in most infections, prevention is the best thing to stop the spread of the infection. Family members must take precautions to not pick up the infection from another family member. Always wear shower sandals when in public showers such as athletic locker rooms or in swimming pools where the fungi grow readily and cross with other strains. Bathe your cat and dog regularly with *Sol-U-Mel* during warm weather. Treat any pet rashes or *"hot spots"* with *T36-C5*, *Triple Antibiotic Ointment*, or *Mela-Gel*.

Bathing is advised over showering. Always put 1 oz. of *Sol-U-Mel*, along with *Moistursil Bath Oil* in the tub. Use a clean washcloth with the *Antibacterial Liquid Soap* or *The Gold Bar*. Cracking or oozing skin should receive a generous amount of *Moistursil Problem Skin Lotion*.

Apply *Dermatin*, *T36-C5*, *Mela-Gel*, or *Triple Antibiotic Ointment* on any suspicious areas of the skin immediately after showering or bathing. Direct sunlight and thoroughly air drying the body after showering or swimming is a great preventive act also. Take *The Vitality Pak*, *Cell-Wise*, and *ProVex* or *ProVex-Plus* with each meal to optimize trace nutrients. Drink 2 to 3 cups of *G'Day Melaleuca Tea* daily.

ROUGH ELBOWS, KNEES OR HEELS

see Dry Skin

RUBELLA (German Measles or Three-Day Measles)

After 14 to 21 days from the time of exposure, susceptible persons will feel tired and may have slightly swollen lymph nodes under the eyes, behind the ears, and in the neck. Other symptoms include the development of a headache, moderate fever and runny nose, and a finely textured pinkish rash which starts on the face and neck, moves to the trunk and limbs, and lasts about 3 days. The virus is spread through the air or by physical contact (see Air Purification). Rubella is much milder in children and adults than *"red"* measles, which not only differs in color of the rash from rubella but displays a painful cough and Koplik's spots on the inside of the mouth. (see Measles)

Women in their first three months of pregnancy who are susceptible to rubella can contract the virus (usually from children) and naturally abort or give birth to developmentally defective and often mentally retarded (congenital rubella) infants. In children up through teenagers, the illness is generally mild. Except for the risk of congenital rubella, some scientists question the risk/benefit ratio of immunizing children. Instead, some still see the wisdom of exposing 5 year-olds to the useful institution of kindergarten where actually developing childhood diseases, in a well-nourished environment, usually gives lifelong immunity. Immunizations offer no more than about 15 years of protection and pose extreme risks. Rubella may be difficult to properly determine without a trained physician using laboratory testing, as some of the symptoms can resemble other illnesses.

Suggested Treatment: Since the active virus can be spread from about one week before to one week after the eruption of the rash, epidemics of rubella sweep through susceptible children quickly. By then the virus has spread throughout the body. Only palliative care can be given to ease discomfort and prevent secondary infections such as pneumonia. Soaking in a hot bath with 1 ounce of *Moistursil Bath Oil* and 1 ounce *Sol-U-Mel* for 20 minutes may help diminish the rash. Chicken soup, *G'Day Melaleuca Tea* and *Vita-Bears Children's Supplement* is the ration of choice. More solid food can be given upon request, which is usually after the rash subsides.

SAUNA BATH

The Scandinavians are right to love the deep tissue cleansing that only sweating can give. Endurance exercises such as racket sports, aerobics, running, and bicycling get the blood and perspiration flowing. Perspiration contains waste products dissolved in water that closely approximates urine in composition. Sauna temperatures of 170 to 200 degrees with moisture quickly open skin pores and speed the process of removing petrochemicals, pesticides, herbicides, and metabolic wastes that resist detoxification within the body. It is recommended for anyone who is not on heart medication, an uncontrolled diabetic, a small child, or pregnant. See the section on Bathing in this book.

Suggested Treatment: Shower or bathe using Antibiotic Liquid Soap or *The Gold Bar* to remove dirt and environmental chemicals from the skin and hair. Drink one quart of water or *G'Day Melaleuca Tea* before entering a sauna. Drink one cup of cool water or *G'Day Melaleuca Tea* for every 5 minutes in the sauna to replace body fluid. Your weight after a sauna should be the same as before you started. First time sauna users or elderly persons should limit their use to only one span of 15 minutes, then shower normally. Veteran sauna bathers can take a cool shower (or jump in a snow bank) then return to the sauna for an additional 15 or 20 minutes for deep cleansing. NOTE: Never sauna alone! Immediately get out of sauna if dizziness, light headedness, or shortness of breath are experienced. Contact your natural physician.

SENILITY (FAILING MEMORY)

Reduced blood flow and lessened oxygen tension within the frontal regions of the brain, as well as accumulation of heavy metals within the brain, are believed to cause premature senility in many people. While scientists have found a strong genetic link in the development of this problem, preventive measures should be taken early in life to postpone or avoid this loss of human creativity.

Suggested Treatment: Avoid toxic environments, old paint, aluminum products (deodorants containing aluminum, aluminum cookware, etc.), heavy fats, and sugar. Ask your preventive-minded doctor to perform a hair elemental analysis to find out if your health is threatened. Take *The Vitality Pak, Cell-Wise,* and *ProVex-Plus* or *ProVexCV* with each meal. Drink 3 cups of *G'Day Melaleuca Tea* each day. Use *ProVex-Plus* to prevent and treat the early stages of this condition.

SCABIES

Scabies are transmittable parasitic infections characterized by intensive itching and secondary bacterial infections. They are caused by the itch mite known as *Sarcoptes scabiei* which burrows under the skin to feed and lay its eggs. The itching is usually noticed most intensely when the person is in bed. The characteristic initial lesions of the burrow are seen as fine wavy dark lines a few millimeters to a half-inch long with a minute papule at the open end. A red lesion occurs on the finger webs, on the under-surface of the wrists, about the elbows and under arms, around the nipple area of the breasts in females, on the genitals in males, along the belt line, and on the lower buttocks. The face is not usually involved in adults but may be in infants. The burrow may be difficult to find particularly when the disease is persistent for several weeks, because the burrow is often obscured by scratching or by secondary lesions. Diagnosis is confirmed by seeing the parasite under a microscope after a scraping is taken from the burrow. The mites can remain dormant in infected bed clothes or blankets for months awaiting a warm victim to bring them back to life. Scabies are nothing to ignore. See the section on Chiggers in this book. NOTE: Treatment of scabies with lindane-containing medications (Kwell) has multiple hazards to children. Nervous system disturbances have been observed and reported in the scientific literature.

Suggested Treatment: Soak in a hot bath for 20 minutes each night with 1 oz. of *Moistursil Bath Oil* and 1 oz. of *Sol-U-Mel*. Apply *T36-C5* to the affected areas each morning and night. Apply *Moistursil Problem Skin Lotion* or *Triple Antibiotic Ointment* to give long term protection against infection. Apply *Pain-A-Trate* to extremely itchy areas. If no improvement is observed within 7 days, contact your natural physician.

SCALDS

Hot water, steam, liquid nitrogen, or liquid propane can produce scalds. Immediate blistering and light colored skin is characteristic. Care should be taken to not dislodge delicate superficial skin. Painful blisters may appear within a few minutes indicating second degree penetration. Loose, swollen skin without blistering is evidence of third degree penetration. See the section on Burns in this book.

Suggested Treatment: Immediately apply cold water to hot water scalds and warm water to cold scalds. Pat dry and apply *MelaGel, T36-C5,* or *Pain-A-Trate* to the affected area. Wrap area with a sterile dressing. Begin treating as a second or third degree burn.

SCIATICA

Spinal misalignments in the low lumbar spine can cause mild to severe pain radiating along the sciatic nerve, which travels down the back of the leg, behind the knee, to the foot. Expert advice should be sought from your chiropractor, as sciatica may be a sign of degenerative disk disease. See the section on Back Pain in this book.

Suggested Treatment: Use a flexible elastic back brace when doing heavy lifting or prolonged bending. Get regular chiropractic checkups *before* a full-blown attack develops. If low back muscle spasms or tension are present, usually after unusual activity, take 2 *Mela-Cal* every four hours until the pain is gone. Take *ProVex* or *ProVex-Plus* daily to relieve inflammation and promote healing. Apply ice for 5 to 10 minutes, followed by 15 to 20 minutes of heat every hour for the first 4 hours. Apply *Pain-A-Trate* to the affected area after each heat treatment. Avoid prolonged sitting. Try to lie down either on your back with a pillow under your knees or on your side with a pillow between your bent knees. To prevent sciatic pain, exercise the abdominal muscles by doing partial sit-ups (crunches) each morning and evening. This not only strengthens the lower abdominal muscle girdle but also helps maintain good posture.

SEBORRHEA

This is a scaly inflammation of the skin that occurs around the scalp, face, and occasionally other areas of the body. Seborrhea usually appears as dry or greasy scaling and is often misdiagnosed as thick dandruff. In the most severe cases, a yellow or red scaling with papules around the rash appears usually along the hairline and behind the ears. It is often found in the ear canal, on the eyebrows, on the bridge of the nose, in the nasal folds, or on the upper chest. Seborrheic dermatitis does not cause hair loss. Infants in their first month of life may develop seborrheic dermatitis, often called cradle cap, which results in a thick yellow crusted scalp. In severe cases, cracks and yellow scaling behind the ears and red facial papules may be present. Genetic and climatic factors, in addition to chemical and allergic sensitivities, seem to affect the incidence and severity of the disease. The disease is more prevalent in the winter when more time is spent indoors and household chemicals are concentrated. Some cases of seborrhea miraculously improve with the avoidance of coffee.

Suggested Treatment: Take *The Vitality Pak, Cell-Wise,* and *ProVex* or *ProVex-Plus* with each meal. Drink 2 to 6 cups of *G'Day Melaleuca Tea* daily for detoxification. Bathe using *Antibacterial Liquid Soap* in a tub containing 1 oz. of *Moistursil Bath Oil* and 1 oz. of *Sol-U-Mel*. Shampoo with Melaleuca *Natural Shampoo* or *Herbal Shampoo* daily. Continue the bathing procedure once daily, but apply *T36-C5* with either *Moistursil Problem Skin Lotion* or *Mela-Gel* after each bath.

SHINGLES

Shingles are caused by the same virus in adults that causes chicken pox in children. Shingles manifests as small, very painful clusters of blisters which form along a sensory nerve on the skin of the chest, neck, face, stomach or limbs. These pink or white blisters contain a clear fluid which may later become pus. They dry up and disappear in about a week, but the area feels irritated for longer.

Suggested Treatment: Shingles can be treated similarly to chicken pox, except for the use of more *Sol-U-Mel* and *Moistursil Bath Oil*, detoxification, and satisfying the increased nutritional need for B vitamins. Take *The Vitality Pak, Cell-Wise,* and *ProVex* or *ProVex-Plus* with each meal. Drink 2 to 6 cups of *G'Day Melaleuca Tea* to reduce virus growth. Add 2 oz. of *Moistursil Bath Oil* and 2 oz. of *Sol-U-Mel* to a warm tub of water. Soak for 30 minutes. Pat dry. Apply a drop of *T36-C5* to pustules followed by *Triple Antibiotic Ointment*. Continue treatment once or twice daily for 6 days. Consult your natural physician if further advice is needed.

SINUS CONGESTION

Sinus congestion can be due to mild infections or generalized irritations caused from allergies, chronic airborne pollutants, dust, grasses, pollens, cigarette smoking, or other chemicals. Often, bacterial sinus infections are caused by repeated use of antihistamines, which dry mucous membranes and lead to severe susceptibility to other infections. Inflammation caused from mold sensitivity or anemia can also be the underlying cause. When frontal sinuses found above and behind the eyes are affected, headaches may occur. Coughing is often associated with deeper irritations in the nasal pharynx and can lead to ear infections in children or nose bleeds in older children and adults. If repeated episodes of sinus congestion occur, the cause should be determined by your natural physician. If bacterial infections are present, the condition is termed sinusitis. When it is not properly treated, pneumonia can result. Prescription antibiotics are becoming less effective against these types of infections due to their overuse.

Suggested Treatment: Drink 2 to 6 cups of hot *G'Day Melaleuca Tea* each day as a decongestant. (Note: For Adults Only. To 1/4 cup of warm *G'Day Melaleuca Tea*, add 1/8 tsp. of sea salt. From a cup, snort the mixture into your nose. Tilt your head back and hold it in your sinuses for 10 to 15 seconds. Expel the mixture through your nostrils into a sink. Blow your nose gently. Repeat morning and evening.)

Dab *T36-C5* directly under each nostril. Breathe the enriched steam from a vaporizer or a bowl of very hot water each morning and night before bed. To do this, add 10 drops of *T36-C5* and 2 *capfuls Sol-U-Mel* to the water. Form a tent over your head and the vaporizer, breathing the aromatic vapors through your nose and mouth deeply and gently into your lungs. Keep your eyes closed. Add 1 or 2 drops of *T36-C5* every 5 minutes for 15 to 20 minutes. Repeat each morning and evening, or run the vaporizer all night. Apply *Pain-A-Trate* on the temples and forehead to reduce pain from the congestion. Repeat every 2 to 4 hours for relief. As long as congestion exists, use *CounterAct Cold, Allergy, Sinus Medicine* as directed.

SINUSITIS

see Sinus Congestion

SNEEZING

Irritations in the nasal pharynx stimulate local histamine production that increases mucous secretion and triggers the central nervous response to expel the irritant. Food or chemical allergies, sensitivities such as hay fever, and viral infections provoke this response. A sneeze is the most efficient way to spread viruses and many bacteria to your family, work mates, and friends. The velocity of air and atomized mucous exiting the nose and mouth approaches the speed of sound! Studies show that particles can be projected up to 20 feet across a room from a sneeze. See the section on Air Purification in this book.

Suggested Treatment: Take *The Vitality Pak, Cell-Wise,* and *ProVex* or *ProVex-Plus* with each meal. A therapeutic dose of *ProVex* (1 capsule for every 25 pounds of body weight per day) may be helpful. Drink 2 to 4 cups of *G'Day Melaleuca Tea* each day. Launder handkerchiefs with *MelaPower* and rinse in a solution of 1 oz. *Sol-U-Mel* per gallon of rinse water. Air dry. For acute sneezing attacks, put 1 or 2 drops of *T36-C5* on a cotton tipped applicator and swab the inside of each nostril. If congestion exists, use *CounterAct Cold, Allergy, Sinus Medicine* as directed.

SORE GUMS

Damage from rough foods, overzealous flossing, or from a tooth brush needs immediate attention to prevent secondary infections and canker sores. Poor dental hygiene or accumulated plaque below the gum line can lead to periodontal infections. See your dentist or dental hygienist without delay. Many health problems stem from improper dental health.

Suggested Treatment: Following an injury, immediately swish your mouth with *Breath-Away*. Follow the printed directions. Apply *T36-C5* to the sore area with your finger or a cotton swab to reduce the soreness. Take *ProVex* or *ProVex-Plus* to strengthen gum tissues, reduce inflammation, and to help reduce plaque buildup.

SORE THROAT

The challenge to our body's immune system comes partly from the air we breathe, the fluids we drink, and the food we eat. Viruses, bacteria, allergens, pollutants, prescription drugs, and overusing our voice can produce a sore throat. Many people get a sore throat if they do not get enough rest. Whatever the cause, proper treatment is necessary to prevent the condition from escalating. Cancer of the throat starts with a mild chronic sore throat with or without a cough. See the sections on Coughing and Hoarseness in this book.

Suggested Treatment: Gargle with *Breath-Away Mouthwash* to reduce bacteria and viruses. Swab the back of the throat and tonsil area with a cotton-tipped swab saturated with *T36-C5*. Spray throat with *Hot/Cool Shot Mouth Spray* as often as needed. If the soreness returns or does not diminish, consult your natural physician.

SORE TONGUE

see Glossitis

STIFF NECK

Muscle injuries or viral infections occasionally result in chronic muscle tension in the neck or torticollis. There can be an involuntary pulling of the head to one side. Every chiropractor has managed this type of problem using manual manipulation, massage, deep muscle therapy, electrotherapy, exercise, and nutrition. See the section on Athletic Injuries in this book.

Suggested Treatment: See your natural physician for specific guidance. Apply *T36-C5* or *Pain-A-Trate* to the affected muscle 3 times each day and one hour before chiropractic care or physical therapy. Drink 2 to 4 cups of *G'Day Melaleuca Tea* each day. Take *The Vitality Pak* with each meal. Keep affected muscles warm. Avoid breezes or too rapid cool-down after exercise.

STINGING NETTLES

An organic acid found in the spines of the mature nettles plant can pack a powerful sting when punctured into the skin. A red, stinging rash results, which becomes quite painful if untreated.

Suggested Treatment: Immediately wash with *Antibacterial Liquid Soap*. Apply *T36-C5* or *Pain-A-Trate* approximately once an hour to the affected area. Usually no more than 3 or 4 treatments are needed.

STOMACH ULCERS

see Gastric Ulcers

SUNBURN

see Burns

TAPEWORMS

Infected meat which is improperly cooked can carry live cysts of the tapeworm. Although the condition is common in Africa, the Middle East, South America, and Mexico, people in North America usually get tapeworms only when raw fish or meat is consumed on a regular basis (Sushi bars). The multi-segmented parasite can grow to be 10 feet long in the lower bowel. The infected person seldom has any obvious symptoms. Symptoms that are occasionally observed are abdominal pain, diarrhea, and weight loss. Occasionally, the person may feel active worms near the anus. Cellophane tape pressed against the anal opening before retiring at night can detect the eggs, which can be seen under a microscope. Blood testing for antibodies or eosinophils can often assist in a positive diagnosis. Diagnosis should be made by your natural physician.

Suggested Treatment: Cooking meat, poultry, or fish to 133 degrees F (56 degrees C) for at least 5 minutes is necessary to kill the cysts. Native Australians have used *G'Day Melaleuca Tea* to eradicate tape worms. Taking *The Vitality Pak* and drinking the *G'Day Melaleuca Tea* with each meal is a good preventive if food quality is a concern.

TEETHING

Tooth bud swelling and eruption through the gum is often a stressful experience for parents as well as infants. Teething often is accompanied by a runny nose and loose stool in 6-month to 2-year-olds.

Suggested Treatment: The cold, mushy consistency of a piece of frozen banana or grape held so the baby can gum it is a quick way to speed tooth eruption. *ProVex*, opened and dissolved in distilled water, juice, or breast milk can give relief from teething pain. *CounterAct Kids Pain Reliever and Fever Reducer* can be used in severe cases where the more "natural" remedies don't give enough relief. Give as directed.

TEMPOROMANDIBULAR JOINT DYSFUNCTION (TMJ)

Temporomandibular Joint Dysfunction Syndrome, or TMJ for short, is an extremely painful inflammatory condition caused by improper jaw development, improper dental bite, traumatic injury to the face and jaw, or muscle tension in neck and jaw muscles.

Your teeth are capable of biting with 5,000 pounds per square inch of force. The jaw joint in front of your ear must also carry this force. Damage to the TMJ disk is a direct cause of the aggravating pain. If left untreated, complete degeneration of the joint can take place, requiring surgery.

If the TMJ joint itself is not injured, the condition is called myofascial pain-dysfunction (MPD) syndrome. This condition is common and is aggravated by emotionally stressful situations. The individual usually has a history of clenching and grinding their teeth. People with this condition will have tenderness to the touch in one or more of the chewing muscles, limited ability to open the mouth, and clicking or "*popping*" sounds are quite common.

Suggested Treatment: TMJ syndrome needs professional advice from your natural physician or dentist. Management may require the use of a night guard splint and therapy by several specialists. In the meantime, apply *Pain-A-Trate* 2 to 3 times per day to the affected muscles around the jaw joint. This is especially effective for MPD syndrome. Get an upper body massage weekly to relieve neck and facial muscle tension. Take *The Vitality Pak* and *Cell-Wise* with each meal and drink 2 to 4 cups of *G'Day Melaleuca Tea* each day. Avoid foods that are hard to chew. Take *ProVex* or *ProVex-Plus* each day to help reduce inflammation.

THRUSH

Thrush is a fungal infection of the mouth or throat, caused by the *Candida albicans* organism. Oral yeast infections are common in persons who are on drug therapy. The condition causes the tongue, gums, inside of cheeks, and throat to have a white patched and swollen appearance. Repeated use of anti-yeast drugs tends to produce resistant strains.

Suggested Treatment: Use *Breath-Away Mouthwash*, as directed, every 2 hours. Brush with *Classic Tooth Polish*. Drink 2 to 6 cups of *G'Day Melaleuca Tea* daily. Take *The Vitality Pak, Cell-Wise,* and *ProVex* or *ProVex-Plus* with each meal. For severe infections, dab *T36-C5* on the area or apply with a finger or cotton-tipped swab. Avoid sugar, alcohol, yeast bread products, cheese, and vinegar products.

TICKS

Ticks thrive in a warm, moist environment. They are often found on dogs, cats, deer, or livestock, and may jump to a human host when given the opportunity. Ticks are instrumental in transmitting several serious diseases, so take great care to watch for them on yourself, your children, and your pets.

Suggested Treatment: Inspect your children and yourself daily when any outdoor activity takes place. If you discover an attached "tick" upon your inspection, cover the tick in *T36-C5*. The tick should soon "let go", and you'll be able to remove it easily with tweezers. Smash the tick thoroughly and flush. Apply *T36-C5*, *Mela-Gel*, or *Triple Antibiotic Ointment* and cover with a bandage for 24 hours.

TINNITUS

Unexplained noises such as buzzing, ringing, roaring, whistling, or hissing are heard by sufferers of this condition. It can be in one or both ears. Tinnitus can be a symptom of almost any disorder of, or around, the ear. It may be caused by low-grade infections, anemia, trauma to the head, obstructions such as earwax, Eustachian tube obstruction from allergies, hardening of the acoustic arteries, tumors, toxicity from chemicals such as carbon monoxide, heavy metal poisoning, many drug reactions, and alcohol. See your natural physician.

Suggested Treatment: If an organic cause cannot be identified, decongestion is the next best approach. See the section on Chest Congestion in this book. If congestion exists, use *CounterAct Cold, Allergy, Sinus Medicine* as directed.

TOBACCO POISONING

The violent effects to the body when tobacco smoke or the masticated juice from smokeless tobacco are consumed testifies to the body's repulsion of such a poison. Animals in nature will not eat the tobacco plant. The dried juice from tobacco has been mixed in water to repel garden and household pests and kill plant fungus. In humans, the symptoms of tobacco poisoning include excitement, confusion, muscular twitching, weakness, abdominal cramps, convulsions, depression, rapid respiration, heart palpitations, physical collapse, coma, paralysis, and respiratory failure. When levels of nicotine in the blood fall below a certain threshold level, a person with nicotine addiction experiences the same symptoms as nicotine poisoning. This level is different for each individual person. In times of excitement, nicotine is degraded and excreted through the kidneys at a faster rate, which causes the addict to crave ingestion even more. Elderly people who have consumed tobacco products for many years show abnormal electrocardiograms and restricted blood flow to the heart, brain, kidneys, pancreas, and extremities.

It is now alleged that the tobacco companies have been *fortifying* cigarette tobacco with extra nicotine, to strengthen its addictive potential. More than 100 tobacco related deaths occur each day. Hopefully, the public outcry for protection will lead to restrictions on this dangerous substance. Chronic exposure to the substances in tobacco eventually breaks down immune response to infections, and thickens the membranes in the throat and vocal cords. The typical deep raspy voice, dry throat, itching nose, and morning coughing fits follow.

Suggested Treatment: Poisoning from tobacco is linked to at least 50% of the deaths from cancer, heart disease, and respiratory disorders. There is no greater single health measure you can take than to quit smoking and forbid the practice in your home or around your loved ones. Like any drug addiction, it must be faced with courage and compassion. If you have the personal strength to stop smoking—do it right now! If you need help, seek professional care. Begin a lifestyle of wellness, rather than self-destruction. Take *The Vitality Pak* and *Cell-Wise with* every meal. Take *ProVex, ProVex-Plus,* or *ProVexCV* daily for antioxidant protection. Drink 2 to 4 cups of *G'Day Melaleuca Tea* each day. Exercise regularly. If congestion exists, use *CounterAct Cold, Allergy, Sinus Medicine* as directed.

TONSILLITIS

Tonsillitis is an acute inflammation of the tonsillar lymph tissue in the throat, usually due to a Streptococcal bacteria or virus. Epidemics of viral tonsillitis occur in the military or during summer camp. Symptoms in older children and adults include a sore throat upon swallowing, and congested Eustachian tubes. Young children will not complain of a sore throat, but will refuse to eat. High fever, headache, and general fatigue are common. The enlarged and often reddened tonsils can be seen on either side of the back of the throat. Repeated treatments with antibiotics tend to produce resistant strains of bacteria. See the sections on Air Purification, Disinfectants and Sore Throat in this book.

Suggested Treatment: Improperly treated tonsillitis can lead to strep throat, rheumatic heart disease, and a chronically compromised immune system. Seek professional help. Begin taking *Activate Immune Complex* at first sign of tonsillitis to strengthen the immune system. For viral tonsillitis, drink *G'Day Melaleuca Tea* every hour. Apply *T36-C5* directly on the tonsils. You may use a cotton-tipped swab. Use *CounterAct Cough Relief Medicine* as directed if coughing, itching, or discomfort is present. Gargle with *Breath-Away Mouthwash* 3 times each day. A positive culture is needed to confirm bacterial tonsillitis. See your natural physician. Until a definitive diagnosis is made, apply *T36-C5* to the tonsils each hour.

TOOTH ACHE

Dental problems are more easily prevented than treated at home. A sensitive tooth, due to root exposure, thin enamel, or cavities can begin aching from things such as sweets, hot or cold foods, or an uneven bite plane. See the section on Abscesses in this book.

Suggested Treatment: For prevention, brush with *Classic Tooth Polish* or *Fluoride Tooth Gel* and use *Breath-Away Mouthwash* after every meal. Use *Exceed Dental Floss* at least once each day and chew *Insta-Fresh Gum* frequently. Apply *T36-C5* directly to the sensitive tooth and surrounding gum to achieve immediate relief and see your dentist to determine the cause of your pain. Have regular checkups with your dentist to maximize the general health of your teeth.

TORTICOLLIS

see Stiff Neck

ULCERS

Overstimulation of the vagus nerve from the brain, too much coffee, rich foods, alcohol, emotional stress, aspirin, or drug toxicity can cause esophageal, stomach, or duodenal ulcers. Acid in the stomach causes erosion of the mucous lining resulting in bleeding, anemia, and fatigue. One out of every 10 adults develops ulcers at one time or another in their life. About one half of the patients with ulcers experience a pain, gnawing, soreness, hunger, or constant empty feeling. The other half have no symptoms, but show signs of blood in their stool. Our modern *"hurry up"* society seems to produce more people with ulcers than ever before. A test by your natural physician for stomach acid production can often identify developing ulcers before any symptoms occur.

Suggested Treatment: See your natural physician and begin following his recommendations. Learn to manage stress more efficiently and take time to enjoy your food. Take *The Vitality Pak* and *Cell-Wise* with each meal. The flavonoids in *ProVex* and *ProVex-Plus* help heal stomach ulcers by reducing histamine secretion and by binding to and protecting connective tissue in mucous membranes of the stomach, so take as directed. Use *This is Fiber?!* as a snack between meals. Drink *G'Day Melaleuca Tea* between meals to revive normal mucous membranes.

URINARY CALCULI

see Kidney Stones

URINARY TRACT INFECTIONS

Almost any normal skin organism is capable of living in the nutrient rich, moist, and dark environment found in the lower urinary tract. Women are more prone to UTI's because of the constantly moist environment of the urethral opening and its close proximity to the anus. If improperly treated, UTI's can progress to bladder infection (cystitis) or kidney infection (nephritis). Fewer than half of the women with UTI's have any symptom of the illness. Tight-fitting clothes, prescription drug reactions, synthetic undergarments, warm weather, inadequate toilet hygiene, or a generally weakened immune system can lead to bacterial or yeast infections in the urinary tract. Usually, drinking enough water tends to prevent or overcome many of these shortcomings.

Suggested Treatment: The best treatment is prevention. Use cotton undergarments. Dry your body well after showering or bathing. Drink enough water and 4 to 12 cups of *G'Day Melaleuca Tea* each day. Take *The Vitality Pak*, *Cell-Wise*, and *ProVex* or *ProVex-Plus* with each meal. Douche as needed with *Nature's Cleanse*. If results are not achieved with these suggestions, contact your natural physician for further advice.

URTICARIA

see Hives

VAGINITIS

Bacteria and yeasts can infect the nutrient rich vaginal lining causing painful swelling, foul odor, colored discharge, and reduced libido.

Suggested Treatment: For acute infections, use *Nature's Cleanse Feminine Douche* morning and evening for 3 to 5 days. For re-occurrences or chronic infections, douche each night. Bathe instead of showering each night, soaking for 30 minutes in a solution of 1 oz. of *Sol-U-Mel* and 1 oz. of *Moistursil Bath Oil*. Avoid sugar. Drinking 2 to 6 cups of *G'Day Melaleuca Tea* each day and 2 to 3 quarts of water per day, along with *The Vitality Pak*, *Cell-Wise*, and *ProVex* or *ProVex-Plus* with each meal, helps build resistance to infections.

VARICOSE VEINS

Enlarged veins in the lower legs are common among civilized people because of standing and walking on flat hard surfaces all day. Chronic constipation and pregnancy also tend to cause circulation back-up in the legs, which leads to varicose veins. Occasionally there is leg pain or discomfort, but usually not. Valves in veins normally prevent blood from flowing backward or pooling. Sedentary lifestyle destroys this check-valve effect and leads to pooling. Varicose veins and hemorrhoids are often found together. Toe action, like walking barefoot on a sandy beach, assists the pumping of blood back to the heart and keeps leg veins and their check-valves healthy. A clinical examination for venous circulation often finds the beginnings of blood clots blocking this natural flow. Some scientists feel that most blood clots plugging brain (stroke) and heart (heart attack) arteries originate in the oxygen depleted veins of the legs. See the section on Constipation in this book.

Suggested Treatment: Elderly people may require specialized care beyond these suggestions. The bioflavonoids in *ProVex*, *ProVex-Plus*, or *ProVexCV* have been known to greatly reduce the unsightly appearance of varicose veins, so take daily. Do not wear tight fitting belts or girdles. Wear support hose ONLY when walking or standing for prolonged periods of time. Wearing them while sitting or driving can cause more circulation problems than it helps. Walk barefoot for 10 minutes each morning in the dew or on a sandy beach! *Sole to Soul Revitalizing Foot Scrub* and *Revitalizing Foot Lotion* can also be used to cleanse and stimulate improved circulation. Maintain healthy regular bowel movements—you should not have to strain at making a stool. Drink 2 to 6 cups of *G'Day Melaleuca Tea* each day and eat one or two *This is Fiber?!* bars each day for added bowel motility.

WARTS

Common warts, also known as verruca, are non-cancerous tumors caused by pathoviruses. Under microscopic examination, the flat plates of the epidermis are seen to be tilted at ninety degrees, growing outward instead of lying flat with the skin surface. Otherwise, the skin cells appear normal. Viral warts most frequently grow on the hands or fingers of children. The elbows, knees, face, and isolated sites elsewhere on the body are less common. They appear most frequently on sites subject to injury. The appearance and size depends upon the location and on the degree of irritation they are subjected to. They can be round or irregular, and are usually firm and dry. Color varies from light gray, yellow, brown, to grayish black. Size varies from 1/8 to 1/2 inch. They may come and go in the same individual in a haphazard way. Infections with the virus may persist as single or multiple growths and develop by spreading from one side of the body to the other. Complete regression is common, with or without treatment. Warts can persist for years and may reoccur at the same or different sites.

Plantar warts are common on the sole of the foot. When they are flattened by pressure, they are surrounded by cornified tissue and may be very tender. They can be distinguished from corns and calluses by their tendency to pinpoint bleeding when the surface is shaved away. Filiform warts are long narrow growths usually seen on the eyelids, face, neck, or lips. Flat warts are smooth, flat yellow brown lesions seen more commonly in children and young adults, most often on the face. Warts of unusual shape which resemble cauliflower or other structures are most frequent on the head and neck, especially the scalp and in the bearded regions. Warts around the moist genital area are often called venereal warts and may or may not resemble warts in other parts of the body.

Suggested Treatment: For isolated common warts, apply *T36-C5* each morning and night faithfully for up to 3 weeks. If the wart is thick and dry, shave the excess away before applying *T36-C5*. *Sole to Soul Revitalizing Foot Scrub* and *Revitalizing Foot Lotion* can also be used to cleanse and stimulate improved circulation. For body warts, bathe in a hot tub with 1 oz. of *Sol-U-Mel* and 1 oz. of *Moistursil Bath Oil* for 30 minutes. Apply *T36-C5* or *Mela-Gel* afterward. Some warts require the added strength of *T40-C3* to disappear. A few warts do not respond to *Melaleuca Oil*.

YEAST INFECTIONS

Yeasts such as Candida albicans are naturally occurring in every human and do not tend to activate the body's immune defenses except in overgrowth situations. They are naturally kept from growing out of control by neighboring friendly bacteria that secrete anti-yeast chemicals.

Broad-spectrum antibiotics given for other conditions innocently destroy these friendly bacteria. When the body is left unprotected by these friendly bacteria, yeast can have a picnic on the nutrient-rich protein found on the skin and sugar enriched mucous membranes. Yeast infections are virtually nonexistent in people who eat simple whole foods. Once yeast infections get started, they must be dealt with in an aggressive, holistic way for best results. Each body site and complicating condition must be addressed on an individual basis for lasting effects. See the sections on Air Purification, Body Odor, Decayed Teeth, Diaper Rash, Emphysema, Jock Itch, Mucous, Paronychia, Thrush, Urinary Tract Infections and Vaginitis in this book for specific details.

Suggested Treatment: Drink *G'Day Melaleuca Tea* and take *The Vitality Pak*, *Cell-Wise*, and *ProVex*, *ProVex-Plus*, or *ProVexCV* with each meal. Avoid sugar, yeast, or mold-processed foods. Apply *T36-C5*, *Mela-Gel*, *Triple Antibiotic Ointment*, or *Moistursil Problem Skin Lotion* to the affected areas.

CHAPTER SEVEN

7

Healthy Home

BATHROOM

BATHTUB - Mix 3 ounces *Tub 'N Tile* with water in a 16 oz. spray bottle. Spray on tub and let sit for about 2 minutes. Wipe clean with damp cloth. For rust spots, apply straight *Tub 'N Tile* to area. Wait until rust dissolves, then wipe away with a damp cloth. For hard water or mineral deposits, use full strength with a soft scrub brush. Initially there may be strong fumes due to the quantity of build up being dissolved, so run the fan or open a window. This problem should disappear very soon if *Tub 'N Tile* is used on a regular basis.

CEILINGS - Mix 1 teaspoon of *Tough 'N Tender* with 16 ounces of water in a spray bottle. Apply on ceiling and wipe clean with damp cloth. For really dirty or greasy ceilings, use 1 tablespoon of *MelaMagic* with 16 ounces of water in a spray bottle.

COUNTER - Add 3 ounces of *Sol-U-Mel* to water in a 16 ounce spray bottle. Spray on counter and let sit a few minutes. Wipe clean with a damp cloth. This will kill any germs that may be on your counter.

FLOOR - Mix 2 tablespoons of *MelaMagic* and 1 capful of *Sol-U-Mel* with 16 ounces of water. Keep this in a spray bottle or mix it in a bucket. Spray or wipe on the floor and mop it up.

MIRROR - Use *ClearPower* (diluted to 1/2 the strength suggested on the bottle). Works great.

ODORS - Use diluted *Sol-U-Mel* to eliminate odors of all kinds.

SHOWER CURTAIN - Mix 2 1/2 tablespoons of *MelaMagic* and 1 1/2 capfuls of *Sol-U-Mel* with water in a 16 ounce spray bottle. Spray on curtain and let sit for a few minutes. Wipe clean with a damp cloth.

SINK - Mix 4 tablespoons of *Tub 'N Tile* and one capful of *Sol-U-Mel* with 16 ounces of water in a spray bottle. Spray sink and wipe down with damp cloth. For rust stains or mineral deposits, use *Tub 'N Tile* full strength. You may need to use a soft bristle brush on stubborn stains. Rinse clean with water.

TILE - Mix 1 teaspoon of *Tough 'N Tender* with 16 ounces of water in a bucket or a spray bottle. Apply and wipe clean with a damp cloth.

TOILET - Pour 4 tablespoons of *Tub 'N Tile* in toilet, let it sit for a few minutes, and then scrub clean with a toilet brush. If you have great build up, turn the water off on your toilet and let it drain. Pour in 2 ounces of *Tub 'N Tile* and let it sit a few minutes, then scrub clean with a brush.

UNDER COUNTERS - Mix 5 drops of *Tough 'N Tender* with 1/2 capful of *Sol-U-Mel* and 16 ounces of water. The addition of *Sol-U-Mel* to the *Tough 'N Tender* mixture takes care of any mold or mildew problem under the counter.

WALLS - Mix 1 teaspoon of *Tough 'N Tender* with 16 ounces of water in a spray bottle. Apply on walls and wipe clean with a damp cloth.

KITCHEN

BRASS - Mix 2 tablespoons of *Tub 'N Tile* with 16 ounces of water. Spray on brass piece and wipe off with clean cloth.

CEILING/WALLS - Mix 2 tablespoons of *MelaMagic* in a bucket of hot water. Use a cloth to wash down ceiling or walls with solution. Let air dry.

COPPER - Mix 2 ounces of *Tub 'N Tile* with 16 ounces of water. Spray on copper pieces and wipe off with a clean cloth.

COUNTERS - Mix 5 drops of *Tough 'N Tender* with 16 ounces of water in a spray bottle. Spray on counters and wipe clean with cloth. For removing stubborn stains, use *Sol-U-Mel* full strength.

CUPBOARD - To clean the outside of the cupboard, mix 1 tablespoon of *MelaMagic* with 16 ounces of water. Spray cupboard and wipe clean with cloth. For the inside of cupboard, add 5 drops of *Tough 'N Tender* to 16 ounces of water. Spray and wipe clean.

DISHWASHER - To clean the outside of the dishwasher, use 5 drops of *Tough 'N Tender* with 16 ounces of water. Spray on and wipe clean with a cloth. Fill only 1/2 of the auto-load cup of your dishwasher with *Super-Concentrated Diamond Brite Gel* in your dishwasher to clean dishes. To clean the inside of the dishwasher, run one full wash cycle with *Diamond Brite Gel* and no dishes.

FLOORS - Mix 1 tablespoon of *MelaMagic* with a bucket full of hot water. Mop the floor and let air dry.

FREEZER - To clean spills, use 5 drops of *Tough 'N Tender* with 16 ounces of water. Spray on and wipe clean with a cloth. To kill mold or mildew, mix 1 capful of *Sol-U-Mel* with 16 ounces of water. Spray on and let sit for 5 minutes. Wipe clean with a cloth.

FRUIT & VEGETABLES - Place fruit or vegetables in a bowl of water containing 1 drop of *Tough 'N Tender*. Let fruit or vegetables sit for about 5 minutes and then rinse clean. This will remove bacteria, dirt, sprays, or wax from the fruit or vegetables.

HAND DISHES - Use 5 to 7 drops of *Lemon Brite* in a sink full of water. For baked-on food, fill container with hot water to which 2 to 3 drops of *Lemon Brite* have been added. Let soak for 1/2 hour and then wipe clean.

MICROWAVE - Mix 5 drops of *Tough 'N Tender* with 16 ounces of water in a spray bottle. Apply and wipe clean with a damp cloth.

ODORS - Use diluted *Sol-U-Mel* to eliminate odors of all kinds.

OVEN - Use 4 tablespoons *MelaMagic* and 1 capful of *Sol-U-Mel* with 16 ounces of water in a spray bottle. Apply and let sit for 5 minutes, then wipe clean with a damp cloth. If it is a major job, use a soft scrubbing pad and straight *MelaMagic*.

REFRIGERATOR - Mix 5 drops of *Tough 'N Tender* with 1/2 capful of *Sol-U-Mel* and add to 16 ounces of water in a spray bottle. Spray the inside and outside of fridge with this solution and wipe dry with cloth.

SINK - For general cleaning, put a few drops of *Tough 'N Tender* into the sink and scrub clean with a soft brush. To whiten or shine a sink, spray with *Sol-U-Mel*, sprinkle a little bit of salt on the sink and then scrub it clean. Watch it sparkle!

STAINS - Soak stained dishes or china in a bucket or sink of hot water containing 1/3 cup of *Diamond Brite Gel*. Let soak for 1 hour. If stain has not dissolved, soak it over night.

STOVE - For minor clean up, use 5 drops of *Tough 'N Tender* with 16 ounces of water in a spray bottle. Apply, let it sit for a few minutes, and then wipe clean with a cloth. For major clean up apply *MelaMagic* full strength with a spray bottle or cloth. Let it sit for a few minutes and then use a soft scrubbing pad to lift off grime. Wipe clean with a damp cloth.

STOVE HOOD (ventilation hood) - Use *MelaMagic* full strength in a spray bottle or on a cloth. Apply and let sit a few minutes and then wipe clean with a damp cloth.

STOVE TOP RINGS - Mix 4 tablespoons of *MelaMagic* in a bucket or sink full of water. Put rings in and let them soak for 5 minutes, wipe clean, and rinse off with water.

TELEPHONE - Mix 5 drops of *Tough 'N Tender* with 1/2 cap of *Sol-U-Mel* in 16 ounces of water. Dampen cloth with this solution and wipe on phone. DO NOT SPRAY PHONE!

TILE - Mix 5 drops of *Tough 'N Tender* with 16 ounces of water. Spray on and wipe off.

TOASTER OVEN - Use either the *ClearPower* or 5 drops of *Tough 'N Tender* with 16 ounces of water in a spray bottle. Spray on toaster oven and wipe clean with a cloth.

WINDOWS - Spray with *ClearPower* (diluted to 1/2 strength suggested on the bottle). Wipe with a lint-free paper towel.

LIVING ROOM

BLINDS - Mix 5 drops of *Tough 'N Tender* with 1/2 capful *Sol-U-Mel* and 16 ounces of water. Close blinds, spray on solution, and wipe dry with a cloth.

CARPET CLEANING - COMPLETE - Mix 1/4 cup of *PreSpot Plus!*, 1/2 cup of *MelaMagic*, and 1 tablespoon of *Sol-U-Mel*. Pour solution into the tray of the carpet cleaner. This works wonderfully! (First test this on a small area of carpet for color fastness.)

Another choice: Mix 1/2 cup of *Tough 'N Tender*, 1/16 cup of *MelaMagic*, and 1/8 cup of *Sol-U-Mel* in 1 gallon of water.

CARPET DEODORIZATION - Mix 1 1/2 capfuls of *Sol-U-Mel* with water in a 16 ounce spray bottle. Spray on carpet and let it sit for 5 minutes. Clean with a scrub brush. Blot with a damp cloth until clean.

CARPET SPOT CLEANING - Mix 2 tablespoons of *PreSpot Plus!* with 1/2 capful of *Sol-U-Mel* and 16 ounces of water in a spray bottle. Apply solution to soiled area. Let sit for 5 minutes and then clean with a soft brush. Blot with a damp cloth until clean.

CARPET VACUUMING - Lightly spray carpet with diluted *Sol-U-Mel* for the most effective vacuuming.

CEILING FAN - Mix 5 drops of *Tough 'N Tender* with 16 ounces of water. Spray on fan and wipe off with a cloth.

CRAYON/MARKER MARK - Mix 5 drops of *Tough 'N Tender* with 16 ounces of water. If you need more cleaning strength, use 1 tablespoon of *MelaMagic* with 1/2 capful of *Sol-U-Mel*. Scrub clean.

DUSTING - On natural and artificial wood furniture, laminated surfaces, vinyl, leather, and paneling, *Rustic Touch Furniture Care* works beautifully. Spray on a cloth and wipe onto dusty area. On all other surfaces, mix 5 drops of *Tough 'N Tender* with 16 ounces of water. Spray on a cloth and wipe dusty area.

FIREPLACE - For the fireplace glass, use *ClearPower* (diluted to 1/2 strength suggested on the bottle). For the outside of the fireplace, use 2 tablespoons of *MelaMagic* with 16 ounces of water. Spray on soiled area and scrub clean.

FURNITURE - For spot cleaning, use 2 tablespoons *PreSpot Plus!* with 16 ounces of water. You may want to test it first on a hidden area. For wood, leather, or vinyl, use *Rustic Touch Furniture Care* as directed.

GLASS - Apply *ClearPower* (diluted to 1/2 the strength suggested on the bottle) to glass and then wipe dry with a cloth or paper towel.

GLASS TABLE TOPS - Clean with *ClearPower* (diluted to 1/2 strength suggested on the bottle). Apply 1/2 tsp. *MelaSoft* and 1 quart water. Spray or wipe on. Dry with cloth towel. This will help keep lint off.

ODORS - Use diluted *Sol-U-Mel* to eliminate odors of all kinds.

WALLS/CEILING - Mix 5 drops of *MelaMagic* with 16 ounces of water. Apply by either spraying on or wiping on with a cloth.

WATER STAINS ON WOOD – Rub *Body Satin Hydrating Body Lotion* into the water stain. Let sit a while, then buff with a soft cloth.

WOOD FLOORS - Mix 5 drops of *Tough 'N Tender* with 16 ounces of water. Spray on floor and then wipe dry with cloth.

GARAGE

CAR CLEANING - For dusting the inside, spray a solution of 5 drops of *Tough 'N Tender* with 16 ounces of water on a cloth. Wipe clean. For windows, spray on *ClearPower* (diluted to 1/2 strength suggested on the bottle) and wipe clean. For cleaning the outside of the car, fill a bucket with warm water and 10 drops of *Tough 'N Tender*. Apply with cloth or spray bottle, and spray off with clean water.

GARBAGE CAN - Pour 1/4 cup of *MelaMagic* and 1 cap full of *Sol-U-Mel* into garbage can. Fill can 1/4 full of hot water and then scrub sides with a soft brush. Pour mixture out and rinse clean with water. Or, use Sol-U-Guard as directed for extra-strength disinfecting power.

GAS SPILLS - Soak a cloth with *MelaMagic*. Wipe up spill. You may also try adding some *Sol-U-Mel* on the cloth as well.

GREASE SPILLS - Pour full strength *MelaMagic* on grease spot and let it sit for 15 minutes; then wipe clean.

GREASY HANDS - Using *The Gold Bar* or *Antibacterial Liquid Soap* works well, or try a little bit of *MelaMagic*. Rub hands together and then rinse with water.

MACHINE PARTS - Mix 2 tablespoons of *MelaMagic* and 16 ounces of water. Spray on the part and let it sit. Wipe clean with damp cloth. If the part is grimy, soak the part in the above solution, then scrape off as much of the build up as possible. Remove the remainder with a stiff brush (natural, wire, or brass) kept wet with the cleaning solution. For small parts, soak a rag in either full strength *MelaMagic* or in the solution, and wipe the part clean.

SAW BLADES - To clean resin buildup from saw blades, shaper bits, or router bits, apply *MelaMagic* full strength. Wipe clean with a damp cloth. Soaking or scrubbing with a soft bristled brush may be necessary. Dry thoroughly and coat with a thin film of light oil (3-in-1, WD 40, vegetable oil, etc.) to guard against rusting.

TAR - Soak a cloth with *Sol-U-Mel* and wipe affected area. This should dissolve the tar right away.

WINDSHIELD WASH – In the summer, use a combination of diluted *Tough 'N Tender* and *ClearPower* to replace the windshield wash in your vehicles. (Make sure to use non-freezing washer fluid in the winter.)

LAUNDRY ROOM

BLEACH SUBSTITUTE - Use *MelaBrite Color-Safe Whitener & Brightener.*

BLOOD SPOTS - Spray clothing with full strength *PreSpot Plus!*. Let sit for a few minutes. Rub it clean under cold water and launder with *MelaPower* laundry detergent. You can also use *Antibacterial Liquid Soap* as a pre-spot and stain remover. It is especially effective on red stains.

CANDLE WAX STAINS - To remove wax stains from linen or carpeting, press a *warm* iron over a paper towel on the spot. Continue to iron until the wax melts and is absorbed in the paper towel. Then clean area with 1/2 teaspoon *Tough 'N Tender* and 16 ounces of water.

CRAYON - Spray affected area with full strength *PreSpot Plus!* Let it sit a few minutes, then scrub to loosen crayon from fabric. Wash fabric with *MelaPower* laundry detergent.

DIRT - Spray affected area with full strength *PreSpot Plus!* Let sit for a few minutes, then launder in *MelaPower* laundry detergent.

FABRIC DYE STAINS - Spray affected areas with *PreSpot Plus!* Let sit for about one minute, then soak in a container with 1/8 cup *MelaPower* for 30 minutes. If the stain is not completely gone, reapply *PreSpot Plus!* and wash in washing machine with 1/8 cup *MelaPower*.

FINE WASHABLES - To launder wool, nylon, or other fine fabrics, dissolve 1 teaspoon of *Tough 'N Tender* in a basin of cold water. Hand wash and rinse in warm water.

FRUIT JUICE SPOTS - Spray area with full strength *PreSpot Plus!* Let sit a few minutes, then launder with *MelaPower* laundry detergent.

GRASS STAINS - Spray *PreSpot Plus!* on stain. Let sit for a few minutes. Soak soiled clothing in a bucket of warm water containing 2 tablespoons of *MelaPower* laundry detergent for a few hours. Wash as normal.

GREASE SPOTS - Mix a solution of 2 tablespoons of *MelaPower* laundry detergent and 1 capful of *Sol-U-Mel* with 2 gallons of warm water. Put clothing in a bucket of water and let soak for a few hours. If the grease spots are not dissolved, apply a squirt of *Antibacterial Liquid Soap*. Rub in with your finger or a soft brush. Let stand for a few minutes before rinsing with warm water. You can also add *MelaMagic* directly to the wash water in the washing machine. It is very effective against grease.

GUM - Pour full strength *Sol-U-Mel* on affected area. Let sit a minute. Rub to loosen up the gum, then wash in *MelaPower* laundry detergent.

INK STAINS - Spray *PreSpot Plus!* on stain and rub with your finger or a soft brush. Let sit for a few minutes, then rinse clean in warm water. Try *Sol-U-Mel* for stubborn stains or dry-clean-only fabrics.

LIP STICK STAINS - Spray *PreSpot Plus!* on stain. Let sit for a few minutes. Soak clothing for a few hours in a 2-gallon bucket of cold water containing 2 tablespoons of *MelaPower* laundry detergent; then rinse clean with cool water. Or, try using *Sol-U-Mel* as a pre-spot, especially on dry-clean-only fabrics.

PAINT - Spray *PreSpot Plus!* on paint spot or splatter. Rub with your finger or a soft brush. Let it sit for a few minutes and then rinse in warm water. This method works very well, but some paint stains are there to stay.

PET ODOR - Launder fabric in *MelaPower* laundry detergent and a capful of *Sol-U-Mel*.

TOYS - Washables: Place all washable stuffed animals, dolls, and blankets in washing machine. Add 1/8 cup of *MelaPower* laundry detergent and 1 capful of *Sol-U-Mel*. Wash as usual.

TREE PITCH - Spray affected areas with *Great Hair Moisturizing Finishing Spray* hair spray. Let sit for about one minute. Wash clean with *Melaleuca Antibacterial Liquid Soap* and water.

WASHER - Before running your first load of wash using *MelaPower* laundry detergent, it is best to run the washer empty with 1/4 cup *MelaPower* laundry detergent to clean out chemical residue. Then run a load of wash using 1/8 cup *MelaPower* laundry detergent. To whiten your laundry load, add either *MelaBrite* or 1 capful of *Sol-U-Mel*. The *Sol-U-Mel* will also deodorize the clothing.

OUTDOOR

ALUMINUM, STEEL, & WROUGHT IRON FURNITURE - Mix 1 tablespoon of *Tough 'N Tender* with 1 gallon of water. Wash furniture down with a rag or sponge. Rinse clean and dry thoroughly. Once a season, apply a coat of automobile wax (If a scratch occurs on wrought iron or steel, apply machine exterior paint with a small artist brush).

AWNINGS - Add 1 tablespoon of *Tough 'N Tender* to 1/2 gallon of warm water. Wet a clean cloth with solution. Wipe awning with cloth until clean and then spray off with water.

BAR-B-QUE - Soak Bar-B-Que grill in a solution of 2 tablespoons of *MelaMagic* in 1/2 gallon water. Scrub clean with brush. For the outside of the Bar-B-Que, use 1 tablespoon of *Tough 'N Tender* and 16 ounces of water; spray on Bar-B-Que and scrub clean with a soft brush.

CLAY FLOWER POTS - To clean moss or algae, spray pot with 1 teaspoon *Sol-U-Mel* in 16 ounces of water. Scrub with a stiff brush or steel wool. Rinse clean with water. Towel dry.

CONCRETE PATIOS - For general cleaning, use 2 tablespoons of *MelaMagic* in 1/2 gallon of warm water. Dump a small puddle of solution on floor, and scrub clean. Spray clean with water hose.

EXTERIOR OF HOUSE - CLEANING - Mix 2 ounces of *MelaMagic* with 16 ounces of water or a ratio of 2 parts *MelaMagic* to 8 parts water. Apply solution by either spraying or wiping on. Scrub clean with brush. Rinse with water.

FIRE ANTS – Spray with *PreSpot Plus!*

GREASE - Mix 2 parts *MelaMagic* to 8 parts water, or apply straight *MelaMagic* on grease spot. Use a brush to scrub clean. Rinse off with water.

HOME/CAR FIRST AID KIT - *T36-C5*, *Clear Defense*, *Moistursil Problem Skin Lotion*, *Triple Antibiotic Ointment*, *Mela-Gel*, *Sun-Shades Waterproof Sunblock*, *CounterAct Extra-Strength Pain Reliever*, scissors, tweezers, Band-Aids, gauze, and a very small container of water (for washing wound).

INSECT REPELLENT - For humans mix 1 teaspoon of *Body Satin Lotion* and 5 drops *T36-C5*. Apply to exposed skin. For outside air, mix 2 tablespoons of *Sol-U-Mel* and 16 ounces of water. Spray into the air around where people are.

LAWN FURNITURE - Mix 1 teaspoon of *Tough 'N Tender* with 16 ounces of water. Spray on furniture and wipe clean with a cloth.

LAWN MOWER - To remove dirt and grease marks, mix a solution of 1 tablespoon of *MelaMagic* with 1/2 gallon of warm water. Use a cloth or rag to scrub clean.

PLANTS - Add 1 tablespoon of *Tough 'N Tender* to 16 ounces of water, or use diluted *Sol-U-Mel*. Spray on roses to kill aphids and other undesirables. *Tough 'N Tender* can even be effective against web worms.

WINDOW/DOOR SCREENS - Mix 1 tablespoon *Tough 'N Tender* with 1 gallon warm water. Dip screen into solution, and scrub clean with a soft brush.

WOOD FURNITURE - To clean dirt from wood furniture, mix 1 teaspoon of *Tough 'N Tender* and 1 gallon of water. Apply with a rag or sponge. Towel dry. For heavy stains, use 1 tablespoon of *Sol-U-Mel* and 1 gallon of water. Finish with *Rustic Touch Furniture Care* and a soft rag.

CHAPTER EIGHT

8

Healthy Pets

Let's begin this section by talking about household chemicals and the health of your pets. If you have not already done so, removing all of the grocery store brand cleaning and personal care products from your home is probably the easiest thing you can do to prolong the good health of your pets. Animals are more sensitive to toxic chemical vapors than us because they are much lower to the ground where the vapors accumulate. Birds are especially sensitive. This is why miners would bring canaries into a mine. A canary would die from any poisonous gasses before the men would be harmed, giving them time to get out of the mine.

ANIMAL FIRST AID KIT

For outings with animals, always carry *T36-C5*, *Triple Antibiotic Ointment*, *Sol-U-Mel*, *Mela-Gel*, and *Moistursil Problem Skin Lotion*, gauze, tape, tweezers, scissors, and water (in a small container for cleaning).

DOGS & CATS

The hair and skin of most animals should not be overly washed with harsh detergents or shampoos. Cats and dogs can develop a sensitivity and produce dry skin as a result of over-washing. However, preventive care during seasonal infestation with fleas, ticks, mites and other insects can be accomplished by proper nutritional support to the animal. Dogs appear to have a particularly high requirement for extra calcium and magnesium. Cats appear to require additional B-Complex, often in the form of Brewers yeast. Both dogs and cats appear to fare very well when treated with *Sol-U-Mel*, *Moistursil Bath Oil*, and *T36-C5*. Optimum nutritional support should be provided based on the individual animal. Your natural veterinarian should be consulted if you are uncertain as to what your pet may need.

ABSCESSES

Abscesses are painful, pus-filled sacks of infection which can occur in or on any surface of the body. Clean the area with *Antibacterial Liquid Soap* and water. Apply *T36-C5* to the abscess. To encourage drainage and drive the *T36-C5* into the wound, apply hot moist packs over the area. When draining, keep the area clean and apply *T36-C5* followed by *Mela-Gel* or *Triple Antibiotic Ointment* 2-3 times per day until redness disappears and the wound is adequately covered with a scab.

ALLERGIES (DOGS)

Just as in humans, allergies in dogs may be treated using *ProVex* or *ProVex-Plus*. For larger breeds, give two capsules per day for the first month, then reduce to one capsule per day. Give smaller breeds one capsule per day and then reduce to one capsule every other day after the first month. Give the capsules to your dog wrapped in a piece of cheese or in the center of a piece of hotdog.

Also for allergies or coughs, apply 1 or 2 drops of *T36-C5* to a cotton swab and swab the inside of the nostrils as needed.

ARTHRITIS (DOGS)

Painful inflammation of the joints usually causes a dog to limp. Some veterinarians are having excellent results using *ProVex-Plus* for arthritis in dogs. For larger breeds, give two capsules per day for the first month, then reduce to one capsule per day. Give smaller breeds one capsule per day and then reduce to one capsule every other day after the first month. One veterinarian claims to have successfully treated 15 to 20 dogs with either hip dysplasia, or some other serious form of arthritis, using this treatment. Give the capsules to your dog wrapped in a piece of cheese or in the center of a piece of hotdog.

BITES AND CUTS

Clean well with water and *Antibacterial Liquid Soap*. To prevent infection, apply *Triple Antibiotic Ointment* or *Mela-Gel* 2-3 times per day until redness disappears and the wound is adequately covered with a scab.

CAT FIGHT SCRATCHES

Cat fight scratches heal nicely with *Mela-Gel* after bathing with *Antibacterial Liquid Soap* or *ProCare Professional Pet Shampoo*. Keep in mind that cat scratches are very serious to humans as many disease-causing germs are found on cat claws. Caution should be taken when cleaning cat litter boxes. For preventing the spread of germs through the skin, use *Clear Defense* to sanitize and kill germs on hands without the need for soap and water.

CUTS

see Bites and Cuts

DERMATITIS

Skin conditions, like rashes, flaky skin, redness or itchiness, should be treated to prevent secondary infections and reduce any stinging or itching. You may need to keep the pet in a clean cage or pet carrier to prevent a contagious condition from spreading to others. Cut the hair around the affected area and wash with *Antibacterial Liquid Soap*. Pat dry. Apply *Moistursil Problem Skin Lotion*, *Triple Antibiotic Ointment*, or *Pain-A-Trate* 2-3 times a day, until the condition improves. See your natural veterinarian if the problem persists.

EARS

For ear mites or to clean ears of either dogs or cats, apply 1 or 2 drops of *T36-C5* to a cotton swab and swab the inside of the ear as needed.

FEEDING BOWLS (CLEANING)

Place 1 drop of *Tough 'N Tender* in each bowl; fill with hot water and scrub clean.

FLEAS

For general flea protection, wash all bedding in washing machine with 2 caps full of *Sol-U-Mel* and 1/8 cup of *MelaPower* laundry detergent. Add 2 ounces of *Sol-U-Mel* to 16 ounces of water, and apply to areas where your dog or cat sleeps or rests during the day and evening. Wash your dog and/or cat with *ProCare Professional Pet Shampoo, Natural Shampoo*, or *Antibacterial Liquid Soap*. If the fleas are severe add a capful of *Sol-U-Mel* to the bath water. It's best to wash your pet outside so fleas won't jump off in your house.

HOT SPOTS

"Hot Spots" and abrasions on the body respond well to *T36-C5* applied frequently to reduce pain, prevent infection, and promote healing. *Mela-Gel* can be applied if drying or scaling results.

INJURIES (SERIOUS)

Pets with serious injuries may heal more rapidly when they get the proper nutrition. Give dogs *ProCare Nutritional Treats for Dogs*. Some veterinarians are noticing a dramatic decrease in healing times when dogs are given *ProVex-Plus*. For larger breeds, give two capsules per day. For smaller breeds, give one capsule per day. Give the capsules to your dog wrapped in a piece of cheese or in the center of a piece of hotdog.

INSECT BITES AND STINGS

Remove stinger. Apply *T36-C5* with a cotton swab to soothe the pain and neutralize the venom. Keep insects off your pet by mixing 15-20 drops of *T36-C5* with 1 cup of water or using diluted *Sol-U-Mel*. Place in spray bottle and shake well to mix the oil and water before each application. Spray the pet before they go outside.

LICE

Isolate your pet to keep the lice from spreading. Wash thoroughly with *ProCare Professional Pet Shampoo* or *Antibacterial Liquid Soap*. Mix 15-20 drops of *T36-C5* with 1 cup of water. Place in spray bottle and shake well to mix the oil and water before each application. Spray the pet thoroughly with the mixture. Brush the mixture in well to soften and dislodge the nits (the eggs of the lice). Let stand for at least 10 minutes. Pat dry with paper towels and dispose of the towels. Dab pure *T36-C5* with a cotton ball to stubborn areas. Repeat daily until all signs of lice are gone. Add 2 ounces of *Sol-U-Mel* to 16 ounces of water, and apply to areas where your dog or cat sleep or rest during the day and evening.

MANGE

Mange is more common in dogs, and is generally caused by mites that bore into the skin and may be difficult to treat. If these suggestions don't work, contact your natural veterinarian. Isolate your pet to keep the condition from spreading to other animals. Wash thoroughly with *ProCare Professional Pet Shampoo* or *Antibacterial Liquid Soap*. Mix 15-20 drops of *T36-C5* with 1 cup of water. Place in spray bottle and shake well to mix the oil and water before each application. Spray the pet thoroughly with the mixture. Brush the mixture in well. Let stand for at least 10 minutes. Pat dry with paper towels and dispose of the towels. Dab pure *T36-C5* with a cotton ball to stubborn areas. Repeat daily until the condition subsides. Proper nutrition is essential, so give your dog *ProCare Nutritional Treats for Dogs*. Add 2 ounces of *Sol-U-Mel* to 16 ounces of water, and apply to areas where your dog or cat sleeps or rests during the day and evening.

PAW ABRASIONS

Treat paw abrasions with *Mela-Gel* or *Triple Antibiotic Ointment*. Apply twice daily as long as needed.

RASHES

see Dermatitis

RINGWORM

Ringworm is more common in cats than dogs and usually appears as a ring-shaped sore. It is caused by a fungus and is contagious, so keep the pet isolated until the treatment is successful. Cut hair away from the affected area and wash thoroughly with *Antibacterial Liquid Soap* or *ProCare Professional Pet Shampoo*. Apply *T36-C5* directly to the area with a cotton ball 2-3 times a day. Be mindful of any signs of sensitivity. Some breeds react to the pure oil, in which case applying *Dermatin*, *Mela-Gel* or *Triple Antibiotic Ointment* is effective. It may take a week or more to clear up this condition.

SKIN CONDITIONS

see Dermatitis

STINGS

see Insect Bites and Stings

SUNBURN

Apply *Moistursil Problem Skin Lotion* or *Mela-Gel* to the area 2-3 times a day. Keep the pet out of the sun as much as possible.

OTHER ANIMALS

FLY REPELLENT (LIVESTOCK)

Mix 2 ounces of *Sol-U-Mel* with 16 ounces of water. Spray directly on the animal.

HAMSTERS, GERBILS, GUINEA PIGS OR RATS

To control odor in or around a small animal's cage or to prevent communicable diseases, dab *T36-C5* or spray a 1:20 diluted solution of *Sol-U-Mel* to the area 2 or 3 times each week.

HORSES

Use *Herbal Shampoo* to wash your horse's coat. The *Herbal Shampoo* has a conditioner in it so it will make it easy to get tangles out of the mane and tail.

To control flies in the stall area, mix 1 cap of *Tough 'N Tender* with 16 ounces of water in spray bottle, or use diluted *Sol-U-Mel*. Apply liberally early in the day. Solution may be sprayed on horse's body to repel flies. Cover horse's eyes.

For cuts: Apply a mixture of 2 caps *Moistursil Bath Oil*, 3 caps *Sol-U-Mel*, 2 caps *Nature's Cleanse*, 5 drops of *Antibacterial Liquid Soap* in 1 quart of water. Spray several times per day to affected area.

For nail puncture wounds: WARNING! If the nail is still in the horse's foot, do not remove until a veterinarian has decided whether to X-ray. The position of the nail near the bone must be determined to predict the outcome of this injury. Horses have very poor circulation in the frog of their feet. Sometimes surgery may be needed! Otherwise, begin soaking the foot in a mixture of 2 caps *Sol-U-Mel* and 1 cap *Antibacterial Liquid Soap* in 2 quarts of warm water for 30 minutes morning and evening. After soaking, apply *T36-C5*, then *Mela-Gel*, and cover with gauze. Repeat for 3 weeks even if horse walks without a limp before this time.

PARAKEETS, CANARIES OR TROPICAL BIRDS

To prevent diseases among birds, use a 1:100 dilution of *Sol-U-Mel* sprayed once per week to the absorbent fodder material on the bottom of the cage. Spray each time the fodder is changed. WARNING! Some exotic birds are sensitive to the aromatic oils in *T36-C5*.

RABBITS

For ear mites, clean ears with Q-tip and then squeeze a dab of *Moistursil Problem Skin Lotion* on a clean Q-tip and apply to the inside of the ear. Massage ear gently to distribute the lotion evenly. To clean a cage, mix 2 ounces *Sol-U-Mel* with 16 ounces of water. Spray on cage and on the bottom tray to clean and deodorize. Scrub clean with a brush. Rinse with water.

CHAPTER NINE

9

Alternative Uses

for Melaleuca Products

WE NEED YOUR HELP WITH THIS NEW CHAPTER!

This chapter is going to be a permanent part of this book in future editions, but we need your help.

SUBMIT YOUR ALTERNATIVE USES

Do you sometimes use Melaleuca products in ways which are different from their intended use? For instance, one person says she uses *Hot Shot* to loosen tough stains on her clothes when she's away from home. The stains come right out when she finally washes them. Another person uses *Clear Defense* for the same purpose. Someone else told me that after she finishes dusting her wood furniture with *Rustic Touch*, she wipes the dust rag over her glass table tops. The residue from the *Rustic Touch* on the rag causes her glass table tops to repel dust better than anything she's ever tried! Did you know *PreSpot Plus!* will take out punch and grape juice stains from countertops? Try it.

These are just a sampling of the many alternative uses for Melaleuca products. There are many others. And not all have to do with cleaning situations. Maybe you have a favorite. If you do, submit it to us and we'll send you 5 copies of *The Ultimate Melaleuca Guide* if we publish your submission. Please send your favorite alternative uses to **RM Barry Publications, P.O. Box 3528, Littleton, CO, 80161-3528**, or e-mail to **uses@rmbarry.com**. Please don't call on the phone as we don't have enough staff to handle these types of calls—thanks. *RMB*

Tea Tree Oil Research

Altman, P.M. "Australian Tea Tree Oil," *Australian Journal of Pharmacy*, 69, 276-78, 1988.

Altman, P.M. "Australian Tea Tree Oil - A Natural Antiseptic," *Australian Journal of Biotechnology*, 3:4, 247-8, 1989.

Altman, P.M. "Australian Tea Tree Oil - An Update," *Cosmetics, Aerosols & Toiletries in Australia*, 5:4, 27-9, 1991.

Anon, "A Retrospect," *Medical Journal of Australia*, 85-89, 1930.

Anon, "Tea Tree Oil," *Australian Journal of Pharmacy*, 274, 1930.

Anon, *Journal of the National Medical Association*, (USA), 1930.

Anon, "Ti-trol Oil," *British Medical Journal*, 927, 1933.

Anon, "An Australian Antiseptic Oil," *British Medical Journal*, I, 966, 1933.

Australian Standard, "Essential Oils, Oil of *Melaleuca* Terpinen-4-ol Type," AS 2782 1985, Australian Standards Association, Sydney, 1985.

Bassett, I.B., Pannowitz, D.L. and Barnetson R.St.C. "A Comparative Study of Tea Tree Oil Versus Benzoyl Peroxide in the Treatment of Acne," *Medical Journal of Australia*, 153:8, 455-458, 1990.

Belaiche, P. "Treatment of Chronic Urinary Tract Infections with the Essential Oil of *Melaleuca alternifolia*-Cheel," *Phytotherapy*, 15, 9-12, 1985.

Belaiche, P. "Treatment of Vaginal Infections of *Candida albicans* with the Essential Oil of *Melaleuca alternifolia*-Cheel," *Phytotherapy*, 15, 13-14, 1985.

Belaiche, P. "Treatment of Skin and Nail Infections with the Essential Oil of *Melaleuca alternifolia*-Cheel," *Phytotherapy*, 15, 15-18, 1985.

Beylier, M.F. "Bacteriostatic Activity of Some Australian Essential Oils," *Perfumer and Flavorist International*, V4, 23-5, 1979.

Bishop, C.D. "Anti-viral Activity of the Essential Oil of *Melaleuca alternifolia* (Maiden & Betche) Cheel (Tea Tree) Against Tobacco Mosaic Virus," (Research Report) *Journal of Essential Oil Research*, 7, 641-644, 1995.

Blackwell, A.L. Tea Tree Oil and Anaerobic (Bacterial) Vaginosis. *The Lancet* 337-300 (1991).

Blamann, A. and Melrose, G.J.H. 4-Terpinenol. *Perfumery Essential Oil Record*. 50, 769 (1959).

Brophy, J.J., et al. "Gas Chromatographic Quality Control for Oil of *Melaleuca* Terpinen-4-ol Type Australian Tea Tree," *Journal of Agriculture and Food Chemistry*, 37, 1330-1335, 1989.

Buck, D.S., Nidorf, D.M. and Addino, J.G. "Comparison of Two Topical Preparations for the Treatment of Onychomycosis: *Melaleuca alternifolia* (Tea Tree Oil) and Clotrimazole," *Journal of Family Practice*, 38, 601-5, 1994.

Carson, C.F. and Riley, T.V. "Antimicrobial Activity of the Essential Oil of *Melaleuca alternifolia* (A Review)," *Letters in Applied Microbiology*, 16, 49-55, 1993.

Carson, C.F. and Riley, T.V. "The Antimicrobial Activity of Tea Tree Oil," *Medical Journal of Australia*,160, 236, 1994.

Carson, C.F. and Riley, T.V. "Susceptibility of *Propionibacterium acnes* to the Essential Oil of *Melaleuca alternifolia*," *Letters in Applied Microbiology*. 19, 24-25, 1994.

Carson, C.F., Cookson, B.D., Farrelly, H.D. and Riley, T.V. "Susceptibility of Methicillin-resistant *Staphylococcus aureus* to the Essential Oil *Melaleuca alternifolia*," *Journal of Antimicrobial Chemotherapy*, 35:3, 421-4, 1995.

Carson, C.F., Hammer, K.A. and Riley, T.V. "Broth Micro-dilution Method for Determining the Susceptibility of *Escherichia coli* (*E coli*) and *Staphylococcus aureus* to the Essential Oil of *Melaleuca alternifolia*," *Microbios* 82:332, 181-185, 1995.

Carson, C.F. and Riley, T.V. "Antimicrobial Activity of the Major Components of the Essential Oil of *Melaleuca alternifolia*," *Journal of Applied Bacteriology*, 78:3, 264-9, 1995.

Carson, C.F. and Riley, T.V. "Toxicity of the Essential Oil of *Melaleuca alternifolia* (or Tea Tree Oil)," (Letter) *Journal of Toxicology-Clinical Toxicology*, 33:2, 193-4, 1995.

Carson, C.F., Hammer, K.A. and Riley, T.V. "In-vitro Activity of the Essential Oil of *Melaleuca alternifolia* against *Streptococcus Spp.*" *Journal of Antimicrobial Chemotherapy*, 37:6, 1177-8, 1996.

Carson, C.F., Riley, T.V. and Cookson, B.D. "Efficacy and Safety of Tea Tree Oil as a Topical Anti-microbial Agent," (editorial) *Journal of Hospital Infection*, 40:3, 175-8, 1998.

Coutts, M. "The Bronchoscopic Treatment of Bronchiectasis," *Medical Journal Australia*, 1937.

Dabbous, K.H., Pippin, M.A., Pabst, K.M., Pabst, M.J. and Haney, L. "Superoxide Release by Neutrophils is Inhibited by Tea Tree Oil," College of Dentistry, UT Memphis, Unpublished 1993.

Davies, P. "Ti-Tree Oil for an Adult with Chicken Pox," *Aromatherapy Quarterly*, 12, 1986.

Elsom, G. "Susceptibility of Methicillin-resistant *Staphylococcus aureus* to Tea Tree Oil and Mupirocin," *Journal of Antimicrobial Chemotherapy*, V43, 427-428, 1999.

"Essential Oils - Oil of Melaleuca, Terpinen-4-ol Type." Standards Association of Australia. Standards House, 80 Arthur St. North Sydney, N.S.W. 1985.

Feinblatt, H.M. "Cajeput Type Oil (Tea Tree oil) for the Treatment of Furunculosis (boils)," *Journal of the National Medical Association* (USA), 52: 32-4, 1960.

Goldsborough, R.E. "Ti-Tree Oil," *The Manufacturing Chemist*, 57-60, Feb 1939.

Guenther, E. "The Essential Oils," *Van Nostrand NY*, V4, p526, 1950.

Guenther, E. "Tea Tree Oils," *Soap and Sanitary Chemicals*, Aug/Sept. 1942.

Guenther, E. "Australian Tea Tree Oils," *Perfumery and Essential Oil Record*, Sept. 1968.

Halford, A.C.F. "Diabetic Gangrene," *Medical Journal of Australia*, 2, 121, 1936.

Hammer, K.A., Carson, C.F. and Riley, T.V. "Susceptibility of Transient and Commensal Skin Flora to the Essential Oil of *Melaleuca alternifolia* (Tea Tree Oil)," *American Journal of Infection Control*, 24:3, 186-9, 1996.

Hammer, K.A., Carson, C.F. and Riley, T.V., "In-vitro Susceptibility of *Malassezia furfur* to the Essential Oil of *Melaleuca alternifolia*," *Journal of Medical and Veterinary Mycology*, 35:5, 375-7, 1997.

Hammer, K.A., Carson, C.F. and Riley, T.V. "In-vitro Activity of Essential Oils, in Particular *Melaleuca alternifolia* (Tea Tree Oil and Tea Tree Oil Products) against *Candida spp.*," *Journal of Antimicrobial Chemotherapy*, 42:5, 591-5, 1998.

Hammer, K.A., Carson, C.F. and Riley, T.V. "In-vitro Susceptibilities of *Lactobacilli* and Organisms Associated with Bacterial Vaginosis to *Melaleuca alternifolia* (Tea Tree oil)," (Letter) *Antimicrobial Agents and Chemotherapy*, Jan 1999.

Humphrey, E.M. "A New Australian Germicide," *Medical Journal of Australia*, I, 417-418, 1930.

International Standard, "Essential oils - Oil of *Melaleuca* Terpinen-4-ol Type Tea Tree Oil," ISO 4730:1994 & 1996, International Standards Organization, Geneva, 1996.

Laakso, P.V. "Scientae Pharmaceuticae," *Czechoslovak Medical Press*-Prague, 485-492, 1966.

Laakso, P.V. "Fractionation of Tea Tree Oil." *25th Congress of Pharmaceutical Science*, Prague. 1,485-492, 1965.

Lassak, E.V. and McCarthy, T.M. "Australian Medicinal Plants," Sydney, NSW. Methuen Australian Pty Ltd. (Publishers).

Low, D., Rowal, B.D. and Griffin, W.J. "Antibacterial Action of the Essential Oils of Some of Australian Myrtaceae," *Planta Medica*, 26, 184-189, 1974.

MacDonald, V. "The Rationale of Treatment," *Australian Journal of Dentistry*, 34, 281-285, 1930.

Maruzzella, J. and Ligouri, L. "The in vitro antifungal activity of essential oils." *Journal of the American Pharmaceutical Association*. 47,250-4 (1958).

McCulloch, R.N. and Waterhouse, D.F. "Laboratory and field tests of mosquito repellents." *Australia Council of Science and Industry Research Bulletin*. 213,9-26 (1947).

McDonald, L.G. and Tovey, E. "The Effectiveness of Benzyl Benzoate and Some Essential Oils as Laundry Additives for Killing House Dustmites," *Journal Allergy and Clinical Immunology*, 1993.

Merry, K.A., Williams, L.R. and Home, V.N. "Composition of Oils from *Melaleuca alternifolia, M. Linariifolia* and *M. dissitiflora*. Implications for the Australian Standard, Oil of *Melaleuca* Terpinen-4-ol type. In Modern Phytotherapy - The Clinical Significance of Tea tree Oil and Other Essential Oils." *Proceedings of a Conference 2/12/1990 Sydney and a Symposium 8/12/1990 Surfers Paradise*, II, 107-104, 1990.

Murray, K.E. "The essential oils of five western Australian plants." *Royal Australian Chemical Institute Journal and Proceedings*. 17,398-402 (1950).

Nenoff, P., et al. "Antifungal Activity of the Essential Oil of *Melaleuca alternifolia* (Tea Tree oil) Against Pathogenic Fungi In-vitro," *Skin Pharmacology,* 9:6, 388-394, 1996.

Oleum Melaleuca; *British Pharmaceutical Codex*, 597-98, 1949.

Olsen, M.W. "Control of *Sphaerotheca fuliginea* on Cucurbits with a 1.5% Dilution of an Oil Extracted from the Australian Tea Tree," *Phytopathology*, 78:12, 1595, 1988.

Peña, E.F. "*Melaleuca alternifolia*: Its Use for *Trichomonal vaginitis* and Other Vaginal Infections," *Obstetrics and Gynecology,* 19:6, 793-795, 1962.

Penfold, A.R. "The Essential Oils of *Melaleuca linariifolia* and *Melaleuca alternifolia*," *Journal Proceedings of the Royal Society of NSW,* 59, 318-325, 1925.

Penfold, A.R. "Essential oil of Melaleuca alternifolia," *Perfumery Essential Oil Record,* 25,121 (1934).

Penfold, A.R. and Grant, R. "The Germicidal Values of Some Australian Essential Oils and Their Pure Constituents," *Journal Proceedings of the Royal Society of NSW*, 59:3, 346-50, 1925.

Penfold, A.R. and Morrison, F.R. "Some Notes on the Essential Oil of *Melaleuca alternifolia*," *Australian Journal of Pharmacy,* 18, 274-5, 1937.

Penfold, A.R. and Morrison, F.R. "Australian Tea Trees of Economic Value," *Technological Museum Sydney*, 1:3, Bulletin 14, 1946.

Penfold, A.R. and Morrison, F.R. "Australian essential oils in insecticide and repellents." *Soap, Perfumery and Cosmetics.* 25,933-4 (1952).

Penfold, A.R., Morrison, F.R. and McKern, H.G. "Studies in the Physiological Forms of the Myrtaceae' Part 2, The Occurrence of Physiological Forms in *Melaleuca alternifolia* (Cheel), (Research on Essential oils of the Australian Flora)," *Museum of Technology and Applied Science,* 18-19, 1948.

Pickering, G.B. "Cedarwood Oil Compounds, Silica Gel Separation and Tea Tree Oil as Nutmeg Substitute," *Manufacturing Chemist*, 27, 105-6, 1956.

Priest, D. "Tea Tree Oil in Cosmetics-The Promise and the Proof," (Technical paper) *Cosmetics, Aerosols & Toiletries in Australia,* Main Camp Tea Tree Oil, 9:4, 1995.

Shapiro, S., Meier, A. and Guggenheim, B. "The Anti-microbial Activity of Essential Oils and Essential Oil Components Towards Oral Bacteria," *Oral Microbiolog. Immunology* (Denmark), 9:4, 202-8, 1994.

Shemesh, A. and Mayo, W.L. "A Natural Antiseptic and Fungicide," *International Journal of Alternative and Complementary Medicine,* Dec. 1991.

Small, B.E.J. "Tea Tree Oil," *Australian Journal of Experimental Agriculture and Animal Husbandry*, V21, 1981.

Southwell, I., Markham, J. and Mann, C. "Why Cineole is Not Detrimental to Tea Tree Oil," *Rural Industries Research and Development Corporation, Research Paper Series* 97/54, 1997.

Swords, G. and Hunter, G. "Composition of Australian Tea Tree Oil (*Melaleuca alternifolia*)," *Journal of Agriculture and Food Chemistry*, 26:3, 734-5, 1978.

Tong, M.M., Altman, P.M. and Barnetson R.St.C. "Tea Tree Oil in the Treatment of *Tinea pedis*," *Australian Journal of Dermatology*, 33:3, 145-9, 1992.

Van Hulssen, C.J. and Meyer, T.M., "Ethereal oils from Melaleuca alternifolia and Melaleuca bracteata," *Inorganic Nederland-Indie,* 8, VII, 84-7 (1941).

Veal, L. "The Potential Effectiveness of Essential Oils as a Treatment for Head Lice, Pediculus Humanus Capitis," *Complementary Ther. Nurs. Midwifery*, 2:4, 97-101, 1996.

Walker, M. "Clinical Investigation of Australian *Melaleuca alternifolia* Oil for a Variety of Common Foot Problems," *Current Podiatry*, April 7th to 15th, 1972.

Walsh, L.J. and Longstaff, J. "The Antimicrobial Effects of an Essential Oil on Selected Oral Pathogens," *Periodontology*, V8, 11-15, 1987.

Williams, LR, Home, V.N., Zhang, X. and Stevenson, I. "The Composition and Bacteriocidal Activity of Oil of *Melaleuca alternifolia* (Tea Tree oil)," *International Journal of Aromatherapy,* 1:3, 15-17, 1988.

Williams, L.R., Home, V.N. and Asre, S. "Antimicrobial Activity of Oil of *Melaleuca alternifolia.* Its Potential Use in Cosmetics and Toiletries," *Cosmetics, Aerosols & Toiletries in Australia,* 4:4, 1990.

Willix, Dr. Robert D. "A Must for Your Medicine Chest," *Health for Life*, 3:5, 4-5, May 1996.

Disinfectant Properties

of T36-C5™ Compared to Other Agents

The following table is a summary of clinical research and is based upon direct contact of the agent with the organism. Standard concentrations were used. This demonstrates the disinfectant ability of Melaleuca alternifolia oil which contains at least 37% terpenols and less than 7% cineol. Please note that although many organisms show sensitivity to certain agents, mutant strains are developing which resist control. Many disinfectants are toxic or cause damage to skin when used over a prolonged time period. For these reasons, a number of these agents are no longer used clinically.

Disinfectant Agent	S	E	B	F	V	C	TOXIC?
Isopropyl Alcohol	K	K	O	P	P	O	
Phenolics	K	K	O	P	O	P	
Chlorine Solution	K	K	O	P	P	P	Yes
Iodine Tincture	K	K	O	P	O	P	
Acetaldehyde	K	K	P	K	K	K	Yes
Mercury Salts	K	P	K	K	K	K	Yes
Hexachorophen	K	P	O	K	O	O	
Quaternary Ammonium	K	P	O	P	O	O	
Boric Acid	P	P	O	O	O	O	
Cidex	K	K	P	K	K	K	
T36-C5	K	K	K	K	K	K	

K = Kills organism
P = Partially effective
O = Does not kill organism

S = Staph Aureus
E = E. Coli
B = Bacteria Spores
F = Fungi
V = Viruses
C = Candida Albicans

Melaleuca Oil

and Healthy Skin

Healthy skin produces many different essential oils to maintain equilibrium with the environment. Each cell of the body has a double fatty envelope that makes up its membrane. This is what separates the cell from its environment. It is the character of this envelope to allow highly selected gases, nutrients, vitamins, minerals, hormones, and water into the cell while excreting wastes with a precision unique to life itself.

When *Melaleuca alternifolia* oil is put in contact with healthy cells, only the Creator of both could describe the complex interactions which take place. Several things are known about plant oils and human skin. Incompatible ones such as oils of Poison Ivy activate a response to flush the substance away from the system. Essential oils are absorbed and mix delicately with the equilibrium and further the harmony of health.

Bacteria have an electrical charge on their surface, much like the electric polarity of a battery. Friendly bacteria have a similar electrical charge to the skin cells they protect. Essential oils, such as found in *Melaleuca alternifolia* oil, encourage the growth of these friendly bacteria. Potentially dangerous bacteria have a lower electrical charge and are destroyed by these oils. Viruses do not carry any appreciable electrical charge and their protective lipid coats are dissolved by essential oils, allowing them to be chemically destroyed by the body's natural defenses.

What do we understand about *Melaleuca alternifolia* oil and this symphony of life at the molecular level? Actually, not much more than what the native Australian people shared with Captain Cook - try it and see what its properties can do for you.

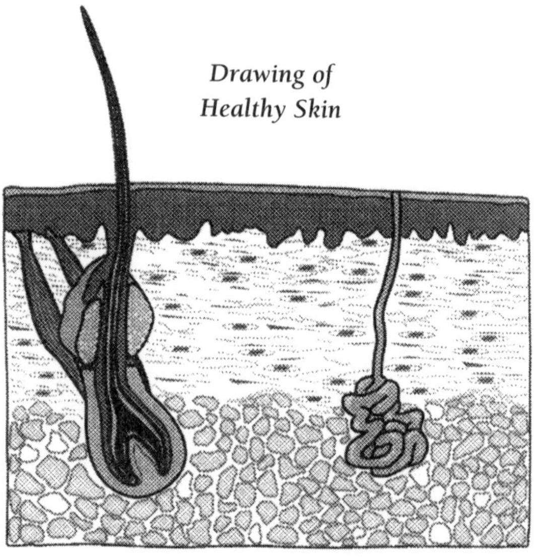

Drawing of Healthy Skin

Technical Information

Although there are over 300 known species of tea trees *(Melaleuca)* in Australia, only one, the *Melaleuca alternifolia*, is known to have substantial therapeutic properties. The most closely related species to *Melaleuca alternifolia* is the *M. linarifilia* that yields an oil that is somewhat bacteriostatic, but is too high in Cineole, a natural skin irritant.

The pure oil of *Melaleuca alternifolia* is known to contain at least 48 compounds. A few of these compounds are not yet identified. A unique compound, viridiflorene, is found only to exist in oil of *Melaleuca*. Two other compounds, Terpinen-4-ol and Cineole, are regulated by the Australian Standards Association to designate therapeutic quality.

In Australia, the minimum amount of Terpinen-4-ol allowed is 30%, and the maximum amount of Cineole is 15%. Terpinen-4-ol is one of the more important therapeutic ingredients in the oil. Therefore, one would want oil high in Terpinen-4-ol. And since Cineole is caustic to the skin, the higher quality oil is low in Cineole. High quality oil should have at least 35% Terpinen-4-ol and less than 10% Cineole.

Since pure oil of *Melaleuca* is entirely natural and the genetics of one tree varies slightly from the other, the quality of oil from one grove of trees may vary substantially from another. In fact, much of the oil that has been distilled from *Melaleuca alternifolia* trees does not meet the minimum standards of quality oil.

Much research still needs to be done to determine exactly why *Melaleuca* oil works as it does and what extract proportion of each of the 48 compounds produces the most effective blend of oil.

In order for any product to give repeatable, expected results, it must be consistent from batch to batch. For this reason, we strongly recommend that anyone purchasing products labeled as or containing oil of *Melaleuca* do so from a reputable firm that has its source of oil and quality of oil well documented.

The following lists the 48 known compounds in pure *Melaleuca alternifolia* oil.

48 Known Compounds of Pure *Melaleuca alternifolia* Oil

1. α-Pinene
2. Camphene
3. ß-Pinene
4. Sabinene
5. Myrcene
6. α-Phellandrene
7. 1,4-Cineole
8. α-Terpinene
9. Limonene
10. 1,8-Cineole
11. γ-Terpinene
12. p-Cymene
13. Terpinolene
14. Hexanol
15. Allyl hexanoate
16. p,α-Dimethyl-styrene
17. (a Sesquiterpene)
18. α-Cubebene
19. (a Sesquiterpene)
20. α-Copaene
21. Camphor
22. α-Gurjunene
23. Linalool
24. (a Sesquiterpene)
25. (unidentified)
26. 1-Terpineol
27. 1-Terpinene-4-ol
28. ß-Elemene
29. Caryophyllene
30. (a Sesquiterpene)
31. Aromadendrene
32. ß-Terpineol
33. Alloromadendrene
34. (unidentified)
35. Humulene
36. (unidentified)
37. γ-Muurolene
38. α-Terpineol
39. Viridiflorene
40. Piperitone
41. α-Muurolene
42. Piperitol
43. (unidentified)
44. α-Cadinene
45. 4,10-Dimethyl-7-isopropyl bicyclo [4.4.0]-1,4-decadiene
46. Nerol
47. 8-p-Cymenol
48. Clamenene

A

Abdominal Distress 71
Abrasions 72
Abscesses 73
Abscesses (Dogs & Cats) 170
Aches and Pains -
see Muscle Strain 133
Acne 73
ADD 80
ADHD 80
Air Purification 74
Allergic Reactions 75
Allergies (Dogs) 170
Alopecia - see Hair Loss 115
Aluminum, Steel, and Wrought 166
Anemia 75
Angina - see Chest Pains 92
Animal First Aid Kit 169
Antiseptics 76
Anxiety 76
Appendicitis 77
Arms/Legs Asleep 77
Arthritis 78
Arthritis (Dogs) 170
Asthma 78
Atherosclerosis 79
Athlete's Foot 79
Athletic Injuries 80
Attention Deficit Disorder 80
Awning 166

B

Baby Teeth 81
Back Pain 81
Bacteremia - see Boils 86
Baldness - see Hair Loss 115
Bar-B-Que 166
Barber's Itch 82
Bathing 82
Bathroom 159
Bathtub 159
Bed Sores 82
Bee and Wasp Stings 82
Benign Prostatic Hyperplasia 83
Bites and Cuts (Dogs & Cats) 170
Black Eye 83
Blackheads - see Acne 73
Bladder Infections 84
Bleach Substitute 164
Bleeding 84
Bleeding Gums 84
Blinds 162
Blisters 85
Blood Spots 164
Body Lice 85
Body Odor 86
Boils 86
BPH 83
Brass 160
Bronchitis 87
Bruises 87
Bunions 87
Burns 88
Bursitis 88

C

Calluses 88
Canaries 174
Cancer Prevention 89
Candle Wax Stains 164
Canker Sores 90
Car Cleaning 163
Carbuncles - see Boils 86
Cardiovascular Disease 90
Carpal Tunnel Syndrome 91
Carpet Cleaining - Complete 162
Carpet Deodorization 162
Carpet Spot Cleaning 162
Carpet Vacuuming 162
Cat Fight Scratches 170
Cat Scratches 92
Cataracts 91
Cats 169
Ceiling Fan 162
Ceiling/Walls 160
Ceilings 159
Cerumen - see Earaches 107
Chapped Hands -
see Dry Skin 105

Chapped Lips 92
Chest Congestion 92
Chest Pains 92
Chicken Pox 93
Chiggers 93
Cholesterol 94
Cigarette Smoking 94
Clay Flower Pots 166
Cold Sores 95
Colic 95
Common Cold 96
Compression Fractures 97
Concrete Patios 166
Conjunctivitis 97
Constipation 97
Copper 160
Coral Cuts 98
Corns 98
Coryza - see Common Cold 96
Coughing 99
Counter, Bathroom 159
Counters, Kitchen 160
Cracked Skin - see Dry Skin 105
Cramps 99
Crayon Marks - Living Room 162
Crayon Stains, Laundry 164
Cupboard 160
Cuticles 99
Cuts 100

D

Dandruff 100
Deafness 100
Decayed Teeth 100
Deciduous Teeth -
see Baby Teeth 81
Depression (Mild) 101
Dermatitis 101
Dermatitis (Pets) 171
Diabetes 102
Diaper Rash 102
Diarrhea 103
Dirt 164
Dishwasher 160
Disinfectants 103
Diverticulosis 104
Dizziness 104
Dogs 169
Drug Poisoning 104
Dry Skin 105
Duodenal Ulcers -
see Gastric Ulcers 114
Dusting 162
Dysentery - see Diarrhea 103

E

Ear Infections 106
Earaches 107
Ears (Dogs & Cats) 171
Earwax 106
Eczema - see Dermatitis 101
Edema 107
Emphysema 108
Enlarged Prostate - see BPH 83
Exercise 108
Exercise Strain 109
Exterior of House - Cleaning 166
Eye Injuries 110
Eye Irritation -
see Allergic Reactions 75

F

Fabric Dye Stains 164
Failing Memory 144
Fatigue 110
Feeding Bowls (Cleaning) 171
Fever 110
Fever Blisters - see Cold Sores 95
Fine Washables 165
Fire Ants 166
Fireplace 163
Fleas 171
Floor 159, 160
Flu 123
Fly Repellent (Livestock) 173
Food Poisoning 111
Foul Taste in Mouth 111
Freezer 160
Frostbite 112
Fruit & Vegetables 161

Fruit Juice Spots 165
Fungal Infections 112
Furniture 163
Furuncles - see Boils 86

G

Gallstones 113
Gangrene 113
Garage 163
Garbage Can 163
Gas Spills 163
Gastric Ulcers 114
Gastritis 114
Gerbils 173
Glass 163
Glass Table Tops 163
Glossitis 115
Gout 115
Grass Stains 165
Grease Spills 163
Grease Spots 165
Grease, Garage 166
Greasy Hands 163
Guinea Pigs 173
Gum 165
Gum Disease - see Bleeding Gums 84

H

Hair Loss 115
Halitosis - see Body Odor 86
Hamsters 173
Hand Dishes 161
Hardening of the Arteries - see Atherosclerosis 79
Hay Fever 116
Head Cold - see Sinus Congestion 147
Head Lice - see Lice 127
Headache 117
Hearing Disorders - see Deafness 100
Heart Disease - see Cardiovascular Disease 90
Heart Palpitations 118
Heat Exhaustion 118
Hemorrhoids 118
Herpes Simplex - see Cold Sores 95
Herpes Zoster - see Shingles 147
Hiccups 119
High Blood Pressure 120
Hives 120
Hoarseness 121
Home/Car First Aid Kit 166
Horses 173
Hot Flashes 121
Hot Spots 171
Hot Tubs 121
Hypertension - see High Blood Pressure 120
Hypoglycemia 122

I

Incontinence 122
Indigestion 123
Infections - see Abrasions, Cuts, and Disinfectants 72, 100, 103
Influenza 123
Ingrown Toenails 124
Injuries, Serious (Dogs & Cats) 171
Ink Stains 165
Insect Bites 124
Insect Bites and Stings (Dogs & Cats) 172
Insect Repellent 166
Insect Stings - see Bee and Wasp Stings 82
Insomnia 125
Itching and Flaking Skin 125
Itching Anus - see Pruritis Ani 141

J

Jock Itch 125

K

Kidney Stones 126
Kitchen 160

L

Laryngitis - see Hoarseness 121
Laundry Room 164
Lawn Furniture 166

Lawn Mower 167
Leg Cramps 126
Leukoplakia 127
Lice 127
Lice (Dogs & Cats) 172
Lip Stick Stains 165
Liver Disorder 127
Living Room 162
Longevity 128
Low Blood Sugar -
see Hypoglycemia 122
Lyme Disease 128

M

Machine Parts 164
Macular Degeneration 129
Mange 172
Massage 129
Measles 130
Menopause 130
Menstrual Pain - see Cramps 99
Microwave 161
Migraine Headaches -
see Headache 117
Mirror 159
Mononucleosis 131
Morning Sickness 132
Mouth Ulcers - see Canker Sores 90
Mucous 132
Muscle Cramps - see Cramps
or Leg Cramps 99, 126
Muscle Pain -
see Athletic Injuries 80
Muscle Spasms -
see Athletic Injuries 80
Muscle Strain 133

N

Nasal Congestion -
see Sinus Congestion 147
Nausea 133
Neck Pain - see Athletic Injuries
& Stiff Neck 80, 149
Nervousness 134
Nicotine Withdrawal 134
Nutrition 135

O

Obesity 136
Odors 159, 161, 163
Osgood-Schlatter's Disease 137
Osteoarthritis 137
Osteoporosis 138
Otitis - see Ear Infections 106
Outdoor 166
Oven 161

P

Paint 165
Parakeets 174
Paronychia 138
Paw Abrasions 172
Peptic Ulcers -
see Gastric Ulcers 114
Pet Odor 165
Pharyngitis - see Hoarseness 121
Pierced Ears - see Abscesses 73
Pimples - see Acne 73
Plants 167
Poison Ivy 139
Poison Oak 139
Poison Sumac 139
Polyps 140
Pregnancy 140
Pruritis Ani 141
Psoriasis 141

R

Rabbits 174
Rashes 142
Rats 173
Refrigerator 161
Ringworm 142
Ringworm (Dogs & Cats) 173
Rough Elbows, Knees or Heels -
see Dry Skin 105
Rubella 143

S

Sauna Bath 144
Saw Blades 164
Scabies 145
Scalds 145

Sciatica 146
Seborrhea 146
Senility 144
Shingles 147
Shower Curtain 159
Sink 159, 161
Sinus Congestion 147
Sinusitis - see Sinus Congestion 147
Skin, Itching and Flaking 125
Sneezing 148
Sore Gums 148
Sore Throat 149
Sore Tongue - see Glossitis 115
Stains 161
Stiff Neck 149
Stinging Nettles 149
Stomach ulcers -
see Gastric Ulcers 114
Stove 161
Stove Hood 161
Stove Top Rings 161
Sunburn (Dogs & Cats) 173
Sunburn - see Burns 88

T

Tapeworms 150
Tar 164
Teething 150
Telephone 161
Temporomandibular Joint
Dysfunction 150
Thrush 151
Ticks 151
Tile 160, 162
Tinnitus 151
TMJ 150
Toaster Oven 162
Tobacco Poisoning 152
Toilet 160
Tonsillitis 153
Tooth Ache 153
Torticollis - see Stiff Neck 149
Toys 165
Tree Pitch 165
Tropical Birds 174

U

Ulcers 154
Under Counters 160
Urinary Calculi -
see Kidney Stones 126
Urinary Tract Infection 154
Urticaria - see Hives 120

V

Vaginitis 155
Varicose Veins 155
Vertigo - see Dizziness 104
Vomiting - see Nausea 133

W

Walls 160
Walls/Ceiling 163
Warts 156
Washer 165
Wasp Stings 82
Water Retention - see Edema 107
Water Stains on Wood 163
Window/Door Screens 167
Windows 162
Windshield Wash 164
Wood Floors 163
Wood Furniture 167
Wrist Pain -
see Carpal Tunnel Syndrome 91

Y

Yeast Infections 156

Book Ordering Information

THE ULTIMATE MELALEUCA GUIDE

(prices are in US dollars and include shipping and handling)

Quantity	Price Each
1-4	10.95
5-9	9.85
10-19	8.75
20-49	7.65
50-99	6.55
100+	5.45

MELALEUCA QUICK REFERENCE BOOKLET

(prices are in US dollars and including shipping and handling)

Quantity	Price Each
1-9	4.95
10-24	3.95
25-49	3.50
50-99	3.00
100-249	2.50
250+	1.95

IF ORDERING BY PHONE

We accept all major credit cards and ship most orders the same day we receive them. Smaller orders are shipped by First-Class Mail or Priority Mail. Larger orders are shipped by United Parcel Service. Orders from Canada are shipped by Air Mail. Call:

TOLL-FREE 1 (888) 209-0510
Local (303) 224-0277
Fax (303) 224-0299

IF ORDERING BY MAIL

We accept checks or money orders. All Canadian checks must be in U.S. funds. We usually ship mail orders the day after we receive them. Smaller orders are shipped by First-Class Mail or Priority Mail. Larger orders are shipped by United Parcel Service. Orders from Canada are shipped by Air Mail. Send order to:

RM BARRY PUBLICATIONS
PO BOX 3528
LITTLETON, CO 80161-3528